POPS

an Autobiography of a Grandfather
By Dan Kovlak

All rights reserved. No part of this book may be used or reproduced by any means, graphic, electronic, or mechanical, including photocopying, recording, taping, or any information storage retrieval system without the publisher's written permission except in the case of brief quotations embodied in critical articles and reviews.

This book is a work of non-fiction. Unless otherwise noted, the author makes no explicit guarantees of the information's accuracy in this book. Because of the Internet's dynamic nature, any web addresses or links in this book may have changed and may no longer be valid. The views expressed in this work are solely those of the author.

Copyright © 2020

Table of Contents

Title Page	1
Table of Contents	2
Preface	4
Acknowledgements	5
Introduction	5
Timeline	6
Cars	7
Christian Business Men's Connection (CBMC)	10
Certified Public Accountant (CPA)	15
Changes Since My Childhood	18
Childhood	19
Churches	28
College	30
Daily Routine	34
Egypt Trip	36
Family:	38
Family Tree	38
Family Physical Stature and Eye Colors	39
Immediate Family	40
Famous People	45
Favorite Books	48
Funny Things	49
Songs	49
Stories (See Appendix 2)	49
Videos	62
Gadgets	63

Governmental Accounting Standards Board (GASB)	64
Golf	67
Hobbies	68
Houses	69
KPMG: aka (Peat, Marwick, Mitchell & Co.)	76
White Plains, NY	76
Stamford, CT	79
Harrisburg, PA	79
Washington DC	81
Marriage	84
Memory Verses	89
Morning Routine	90
Nichols Engineering	92
Non-profit Organizations	94
Number Facts	97
Pets	98
Publications	100
Quotes (Se Appendix 3)	101
Restaurants, Amusement Parks, & Museums	103
Salvation	105
Sovereign Grace	111
Spinocerebellar Ataxia (See Appendix 1)	112
Therapies	117
Travel	119
Worldwide Pandemic of 2020	124
Appendix 1 Spinocerebellar ataxia	129
Appendix 2 Table Of Contents - Funny Stories	134
Appendix 3 Table Of Contents Quotes	136
Appendix 4 CBMC Connector News Article	137

Preface

I titled this book "POPS, an autobiography of a grandfather" because my grandchildren call me 'Pops." I seriously considered another title "1 in 5 Million." The reason why I considered the title "1 in 5 Million" was because it explains how my life has been unique. Every person who has ever been born is a unique person. One characteristic in my life makes me literally 1 in 5 million.

In 2010, I was diagnosed with a hereditary, degenerative, nerve disease. The name of the disease is SCA. That stands for Spinocerebellar Ataxia. It is a rare disease where part of the brain (cerebellum) gradually degenerates. As this occurs, motor skills deteriorate. With the type of SCA that I have, this process takes approximately 20 years.

In order to get this disease, you have to inherit an SCA gene from one of your parents. Approximately 150,000 people in the United States have this disease. I have two cousins with this disease and one second cousin. Researchers have found that there are approximately 40 different types of SCA. I have type 1 and type 8. That means I inherited type 1 from one of my parents and type 8 from the other parent. My father was dead when I was diagnosed, so he could not be tested to find out what type he had. However, my mother was still alive. She was tested and it was determined that she had type 8. She had no symptoms. The cousins that are exhibiting SCA characteristics all have SCA type 1 and they are all on my father side. Therefore, I must have received the SCA type 1 gene from my father and type 8 from my mother. That is very rare. None of my neurologists have ever seen anyone with two types of SCA. In fact, many neurologists have never seen one person with one type of SCA.

Being a numbers guy (I spent my entire career as a certified public accountant.), I realized that having both parents with this rare disease would result in 1 in 5.4 million people.

Acknowledgements

Special thanks goes to my brother Vinny for fact checking much of this book and to Charlie Liebert who led me through the book publishing process.

Introduction

I decided to write this book primarily for my grandchildren. However, if anyone else can benefit from this book, I will be happy. I did not know my grandparents well; so, I would like to have my grandchildren learn a little about me from this book.

This book began with the ideas that I had to express at the speech therapy I took in February 2018. In order to judge my speech, the therapists asked me several interesting questions. I realized that the answers were also very interesting, and I should share these with others.

While reading a book simultaneously with several of my grown daughters, we realized that short chapters are more fun, and they give the reader a feeling of accomplishment when a chapter is completed. Therefore, each of these chapters is relatively short.

For ease of reading, I have decided to put most of the chapters in alphabetical order. This will allow the reader to read about my life by topic rather than chronologically. As a result of this format, there are some areas of repetition.

With this book, I would like to give God the glory for a wonderful life. I would like to share this wonderful life with others.

Finally, I know writing a book is not an impossible task because several of my friends have done that already. One of my author friends tells the story that his "book is a million seller." He goes on to say that "1 million copies are in his cellar." LOL

Enjoy the book!

Timeline

1954 - 1972	Childhood
1954 - Present	Changes Since My Childhood
1954 - Present	Churches
1971 - Present	Travel
1972 – 1983	Colleges
1973 – 1976	Nichols Engineering
1973 - Present	Marriage
1973 - Present	Salvation
1973 - Present	Sanctification
1976 - 1980	KPMG, White Plains, NY
1979 – 2012	Certified Public Accountant
1980 - 1987	KPMG, Stamford, CT
1984 - 1986	Governmental Accounting Standards Board (GASB)
1987 - 2002	KPMG, Harrisburg, PA
1999 - Present	Christian Business Men's Connection
2002 – 2012	Sovereign Grace Church
2002 - 2012	KPMG, Washington DC
2007	Egypt Trip
2010 - Present	Spinocerebellar Ataxia
2012 – Present	Retired
2020 – Present	Worldwide Pandemic of 2020

Cars

This section of the book was written to bring back fond memories of many of the car trips we took with our daughters. These were local trips as well as vacations. This will also bring back memories for the girls when they were learning how to drive. The cars that we have owned over the years follow:

Dan's Cars

Black 1973 Nova

Blue 1976 Chevette

Light blue 1986 Chrysler Calais

Black 1991 Cadillac Sedan Deville

Sea Mist Green 1996 Cadillac Sedan Deville

In 2009, this car had relatively low mileage, and it had very little wear. It looked brand new even though I had it for around ten years. Its market value was very low, so I sold it to a dealer in the "cash for clunkers" program. This federal program aimed to get high polluting older cars off the road in order to have people purchase more energy-efficient vehicles. We bought a new Saturn SUV for our daughter Kelly to drive while at Liberty University in Lynchburg, VA. (It broke my heart to call this beautiful, well-kept car a "clunker.")

Gold 2002 Jeep Grand Cherokee

Green 2002 Jeep Liberty

Black 2013 Acura XLS hybrid

Navy blue 2013 Tesla Model S

Metallic titanium 2015 Tesla Model S with Autopilot

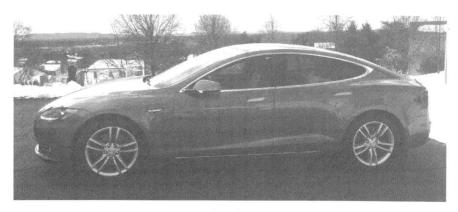

Tesla

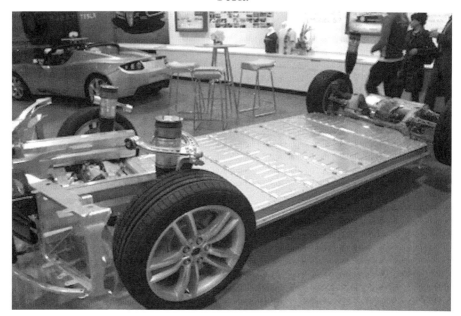

Tesla Battery

I took two relatively long Tesla trips to Toledo, Ohio, to visit my daughter, Danielle Wilson and her family. It is about 420 miles one way from Mechanicsburg, PA to Toledo, OH. The first trip was without Autopilot. The second trip was with Autopilot. Even with Autopilot, the journey was challenging on the winding, mountainous roads on Route 76 near Pittsburgh.

The nice thing was that the trips required no gasoline in the Tesla. The charging stations were free. They were not far out of the way. Rather than going all the way to Toledo, the goal was to go to the next charging station. So, several goals were accomplished with one trip. The stations were about 150 miles apart. The Tesla could go about 260 miles when fully charged, so it had plenty of miles left when I reached the next charging station. The charging stations were all very close to restaurants, Starbucks, or other eateries.

Autopilot steers the car as long as there are lines in the road, and it also has cruise control, which slows the Tesla to a stop if the vehicle in front of you slows down or stops.

Terri's Cars

Black 1963 Chevy Bel Air (Uncle Bob's Bomb)

Black 1973 Nova

Dark Gray Plymouth minivan

Blue and white 1988 full-size Chevy Conversion Van

Green 1997 Saturn

Silver 1990 Mazda Miata

Green 2002 Jeep Liberty

Maroon 2003 Chrysler minivan

Silver 2013 Toyota minivan

Christian Business Men's Connection (CBMC)

I began attending Christian Business Men's Connection (CBMC) meetings around 1999. We held weekly meetings at the YMCA in Mechanicsburg, PA. There were about 6 participants. I was a member of CBMC for several years.

When I moved to Maryland In 2002, I could not find a CBMC group that fit my work schedule. They formed one around 2009 in Gaithersburg, where I lived. I started attending meetings of this group until I moved back to PA in 2012. In 2013, I began attending the Mechanicsburg CBMC group in Pennsylvania.

I have gone to the International CBMC conference in Orlando and The President's Council meetings in Amelia Island, Florida, The Homestead in West Virginia, and in Atlanta, Georgia. I have also gone to area meetings of CBMC in Gettysburg twice and the Maritime Conference Center near Baltimore.

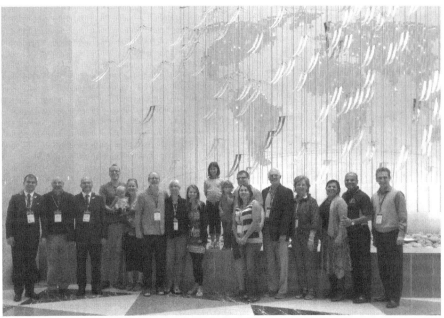

CBMC International Conference - Orlando

CBMC has an excellent website and tremendous resources, which includes the electronic Operation Timothy discipleship booklets. These booklets are available in electronic format (EOT). I have had several life-changing Operation Timothy discipleship relationships over the years. I have also made some lifelong Christian friends/brothers through CBMC, both locally and nationally.

I tried to start a CBMC group in Ponte Vedra, FL, in 2020. I held the meetings of the new group for three weeks with no one else attending. Then Covid 19 came upon us, and I deferred the start of our new group.

I distributed the following information to Christian men in the area before our first meeting. I also verbally explained how CBMC works.

****

CBMC - Brief Background and History

CBMC is an international Christian organization of men who meet weekly to pray, study God's word, and disciple other Christian men.

I am from Pennsylvania and attend CBMC meetings there. However, this winter, I am spending several months in Ponte Vedra, FL. Since we do not have a CBMC group in Ponte Vedra, I thought we could start one.

I have been involved with CBMC for around 20 years. CBMC is nondenominational. The meetings are usually from 6:30 AM to 7:30 AM. (We can be flexible regarding the time and location.)

CBMC is a movement of business and professional men who believe God has called them to take Christ to the marketplace. It was started in Chicago in the 1930s.

We have members other than from businesses such as government agencies, academia, religious and other non-profit organizations, and retirees.

There are no dues; voluntary contributions to the headquarters in Chattanooga only.

Resources:

Operation Timothy materials (hard copy 3 volume set and Leaders Guide. Electronic OT - free). OT discipleship meetings are Important.,

Monday Manna website - CBMC Canada,

Marketplace Ambassador course - 10 weeks,

Living Proof videos,   Connect 3 meetings,

Coaching course - 10 weeks,   More on the website.

10 Most Wanted cards,

This is not solely a men's bible study, but instead focuses on helping each other be fruitful in our endeavors to bring other men to Christ with a component of healthy accountability.

Key Verses:

Proverbs 27:17, *Iron sharpens iron, and one man sharpens another.*

2 Cor. 5:20, *Therefore, we are ambassadors for Christ, God making his appeal through us. We implore you on behalf of Christ, be reconciled to God.*

Monday morning at 6:30 is a great way to start the workweek (with other Christian men.)

Agenda for meetings:

Prayer 10-15 minutes; Read, Discuss, Fellowship – 45-50 minutes. End in prayer. Leave at 7:30 sharp.

First Meeting: Monday, February 24, 2020, 6:30 AM, at the Nocatee Town Center Panera.

Websites. www.marketplaceambassador.com   www.cbmc.com

Handouts

10 Most Wanted cards

OT, three books: Tables of Contents (also on-line for free with hyperlinks to Bible verses.)

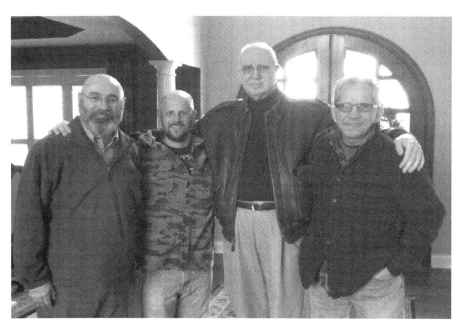

CBMC Men

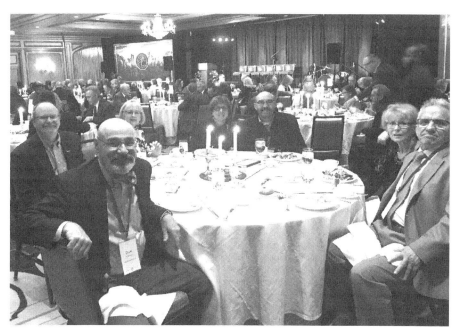

CBMC Dinner - Atlanta, GA

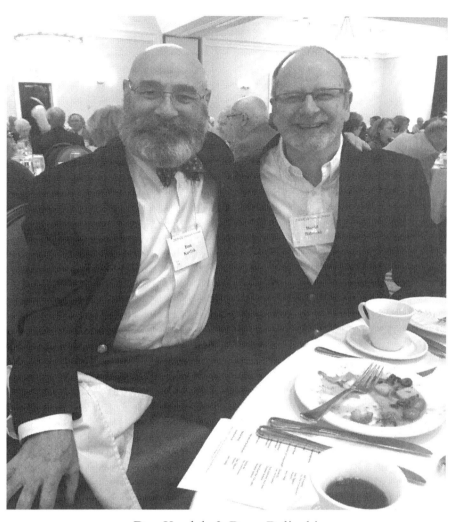

Dan Kovlak & Dave Balinski

Contact Info

Dan Kovlak   301-300-7245.   dlkovlak@gmail.com

CBMC Article

Appendix 4 contains an article from the CBMC Connector newsletter titled; "Dan Kovlak: Being introduced to CBMC was 'TREMENDOUS' from the start."

Certified Public Accountant (CPA)

As I was growing up, my father was an auto mechanic, and my mother was a trained nurse/stay at home mom. When I was in sixth grade, my father let me work in his garage with him temporarily. Through that experience, I learned that I did not want to be an auto mechanic for my profession.

I always wanted to go into "business." Therefore, my goal was to get a bachelor of science in business administration degree (BSBA) with a finance major. However, after one year, I felt it would be wise to change my major to "accounting."

I got good grades in college and was able to take a job as a certified public accountant trainee in the White Plains office of Peat, Marwick, Mitchell & Co. I was rejected by two of the other "Big Eight" firms that interviewed at the University of New Haven.

I took the CPA exam three times before I passed all four parts. At that time, in order to be a certified public accountant in Connecticut, you needed two years of experience, a college degree, and to pass the CPA exam. Fortunately, I passed the CPA exam within the two years, so I became certified in January 1979 in Connecticut. When I took the CPA exam, it was only offered in May and November of each year. It was a two and ½ day exam. It was not computerized. The participants could not even use a calculator at that time. Subsequent to that, I received my CPA certification in New York state. When I transferred to Pennsylvania, I became certified in Pennsylvania. When I moved to the Washington DC office of KPMG (formerly Peat Marwick) in 2002, I had to be certified in Washington, DC, Virginia, and Maryland. I had to be certified in those jurisdictions because I had clients there and I worked on audits there. During my career, almost all the states passed "mobility" laws. This allows CPAs to work temporarily in different states without getting certified in that state.

During my years as a CPA, I joined the Pennsylvania Institute of Certified Public Accountants. I was on their board of directors for several years. I was very active in the PICPA, serving as the Government Committee chairman for several years.

Since I was on their board for several years, I was elected President from 2002 through 2003. However, since I transferred to the DC area at that time, I never served my term as President of the Pennsylvania Institute of CPAs. I have made lifelong friendships through that organization. Ron Rogozinski was the President of the PICPA when I was the 1st Vice President. We are still very close friends.

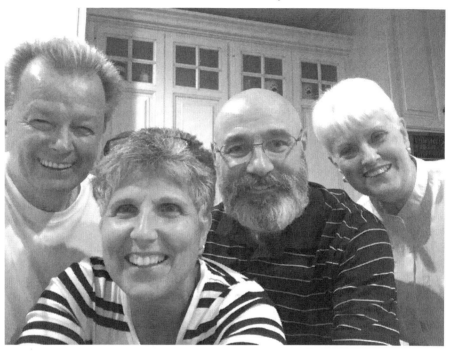

Ron, Terri, Dan, & Mary

When I moved to the DC area, I joined the Greater Washington Society of CPAs. I also served on its board of directors for several years and on its committee to help DC pass "mobility" legislation.

God blessed me with a great career as a CPA. I traveled the right amount of time. When I would travel, I liked to bring little gifts back for the rest of the family.

My clients were great, my co-workers were great, and my peers were great. I had some great mentors that helped guide my career. John Azzariti taught me numerous managerial skills, including client entertainment. He became a close personal friend, and our families became close friends. John R. (Jack) Miller was KPMG's Vice Chairman in charge of the government practice. He was the partner that encouraged me to do a 2-year Practice Fellowship at the Governmental Accounting Standards Board (GASB). He was also integral in my transfer from the Stamford, CT office of Peat Marwick to the Harrisburg office to audit the financial statements of the Commonwealth of PA. They were both instrumental in my admission to the KPMG partnership in 1987.

Since our accounting firm was relatively conservative, very few people had facial hair. Throughout my career, I was one of the few that had a mustache. When I retired, I grew a beard. I started shaving my head in 2001 because I was going bald, and I thought the shaved head was neater.

Virtually no one wore bow ties to work. When I went to special events in the last few years of my career, I would wear a bow tie. (I always wore "self-tie" bow ties, not the pre-tied ones.) Now that I am retired, I wear bow ties when I go to Lions Club meetings and special events.

When I began my CPA career, we were required to wear a suit to work, even if you worked in the office. (Sports jackets were not allowed.) Around 1990, we were allowed to wear business casual dress. On Fridays, we could wear jeans. You would have to dress following your client's dress code if you worked at a client location. When I transferred to the Washington DC office, most of my clients were Federal agencies. Most of these agencies required suits. When I was in DC, my primary attire was suits and neckties. Throughout my career, I wore cuff links and French cuff shirts. I also always carried Listermints with me, so my breath would be fresh when I talked to other people.

Charlie "Tremendous" Jones used to say that "5 years from now you will be the same person you are now except for the people you meet and the books you read." This is so true. You meet a lot of people as a CPA (auditor).

Changes Since My Childhood

I was born in 1954. The world has changed a lot since my childhood. I'm sure it will continue to change. Here are some of the changes in the last 60+ years.

Alexa Devices	Facebook	Podcasts
Apple Watches	Facetime	Printers
Audio Books	Flatscreen TVs	Seatbelts
Cable TV	Google	Smartphones
Cell phones	GPSs	Streaming TV
Colored TVs	HD TVs	Video games
Computers	iPads	Wikipedia
Digital Cameras	Laptops	You Tube
Electric/hybrid cars	Microwave Ovens	

The following corporations are new since my birth: Apple, Amazon, Tesla, Wendy's, McDonald's, Burger King, Taco Bell, Chik-fil-A, Walmart, Sam's Club, Costco, BJ's, Google, and Facebook.

One thing that was done away with since my youth was the military draft. In my father's generation, all men were drafted into the military for two years. The draft ended in 1973. Now, the military is entirely voluntary. Since I was 18 before 1973, I had to register for the draft. I was in college when the draft ended.

My brother and I were included in the draft lottery when we were 18 (before the draft ended.) The higher your draft lottery number, the less likely you would be drafted into the military.

For the year of my birth, my lottery number came out to be number 365. My brother was a year earlier. He was number 11 that year. (A high likelihood that he would have been drafted if he was not in college at the time.) I used to tell people that because my draft lottery number was 365, the military would draft women and children before me. LOL.

Childhood

I grew up at 195 Holmes St., Stratford, CT. I have very good memories of my childhood.

While I was a child, we had four dogs at different times. The first dog was named Suzy. We had her from when I was 5 until I was 12. Then we got Amos. We only had him a few months, and he got hit by a car. Then we got Becky. Becky had some puppies, and we kept one of the puppies - Winnie. We had Winnie and Becky until I grew up.

In our neighborhood, there were lots of kids to play with that were my age. They were Peter, Teddy, Donald, Chucky, David, and my brother Vinny (who is 20 months older than me.)

My mother's best friend was Edith Friedman. She lived down the street. She would walk over to our house and sit in the living room to talk and smoke cigarettes with my mother. She was about 30 years older than my mother. Her husband's name was Jack. They had no children of their own, but they were very nice to us. My mother smoked for over 50 years. She gave up smoking, cold turkey, at around age 75 because she felt cigarettes were getting too expensive.

When I was a child, I liked to play baseball, pinball, the player piano, and HO race cars. My brother and I also took accordion lessons for about three years. He was much better at that than I was. We would also play Monopoly with friends in our enclosed front porch. Sometimes, one game would last for several days. For many years, my father would make many bottles of home-made root beer soda.

In my early childhood, my parents would go bowling. I learned how to bowl at an early age. I also bowled on the high school bowling team, and as adults, Terri and I bowled on the Carlisle Country Club bowling league.

Soccer was not popular at that time. Our parents would not allow us to play football because they felt it was too dangerous. Although basketball was somewhat popular at the time, neither my brother nor I played organized basketball.

We rode our bikes a lot and painted them a lot. In the 1960s, the bicycles were called Sting-rays. They had long "banana seats" and high-rise handlebars.

I had a paper route for several years when I was around 13 years old. I learned the value of hard work, responsibility, commitment, and business management. I would save my money and use it to go bowling or travel to downtown Bridgeport with my brother and friends. In those days, I could get a large slice of pizza for $.35. Now it costs about ten times that!

I had several accidents on my bicycle. One time, my baseball shoes were tied to my handlebars. They got loose and got into the front wheel of my bike. They immediately acted as a front brake, and I got thrown off of the bike. A stranger saw it happen and brought me home.

At around age 10, I had another bicycle accident. I broke my two front teeth. They were broken until I was age 35 when I had them crowned.

The Sterbin family, from Wisconsin, would visit us almost every year. Frank Sterbin, Sr. was my mother's brother. They had six kids that were around our age. They would come to visit almost every summer. We had fun playing with them. We visited them when we took our cross-country trip in 1971 in my father's Chevy Suburban. Wisconsin was one of our last stops.

Aunt Hon (Helen) and Uncle Bob would come over to visit us almost every Wednesday night during my childhood. Aunt Hon was like a grandmother. She was my father's sister and had no children of her own. She was very kind to us. She was born in 1912 and died in 1988. My father was born in 1930 and died in 2006. She lived for 76 years and two days. My father lived for 76 years and three days.

My father was a hard worker. He had his own auto repair shop, Vinny's Garage, from 1962 to 1984. He went to work at 6 AM every day and got home at 5 PM. He worked Saturday mornings but did not work on Sundays.

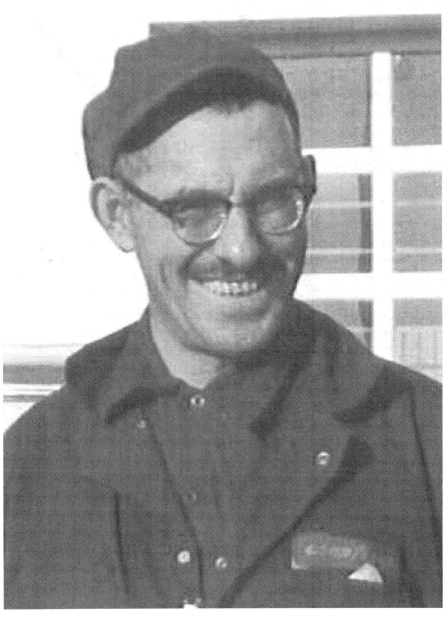

Grandpa K. at Vinny's Garage

His brother, Donny, worked with him most of those years. Donnie was born in 1939 and died in 2010. He was 71 years old. My father and Uncle Donny both had Spinocerebellar Ataxia (SCA). My father's older brother, Leonard, also had SCA.

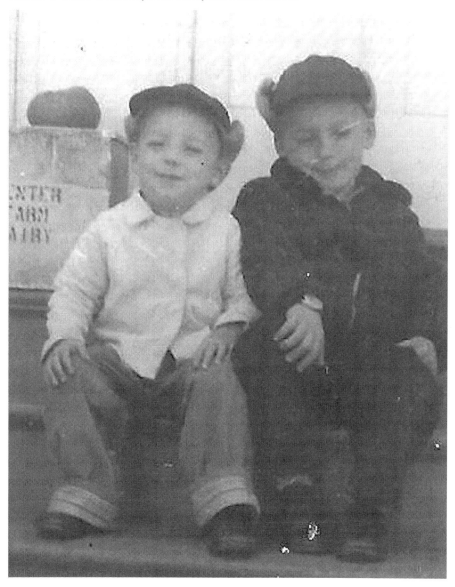

Kovlak Brothers 1959 (Danny & Vinny)

My father could fix almost anything (unlike me). When Jennifer was around three years old, her balloon broke. She said, "Let's bring it to Grandpa; he can fix anything." He was very generous.

My mother was a stay-at-home mom. She was a registered nurse and worked several years before she had children. She would help us with our homework when we were children. She cooked supper every night. It was ready when my father got home from work at 5 PM.

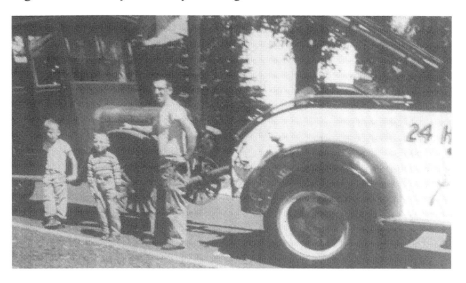

Vinny Jr., Danny, and Papa

There were very few restaurants to go to in those days, so we ate out very seldomly. My mother was very frugal and a wise money manager. She did all of the accounting for my father's business. This was for over 20 years. Both parents instilled good values in my brother and me. These included hard work, honesty, getting a good education, being organized, respecting authority, being frugal, and being generous. Another thing I learned from my father was to put the date that I acquired an item on the box or the item to determine how long a particular item would last. (I still do that.)

My mother was very witty until the day she died. She loved to write poetry when she was young. She was very good at knitting and crocheting. She taught Terri these skills. Neither my father nor my mother drank alcohol.

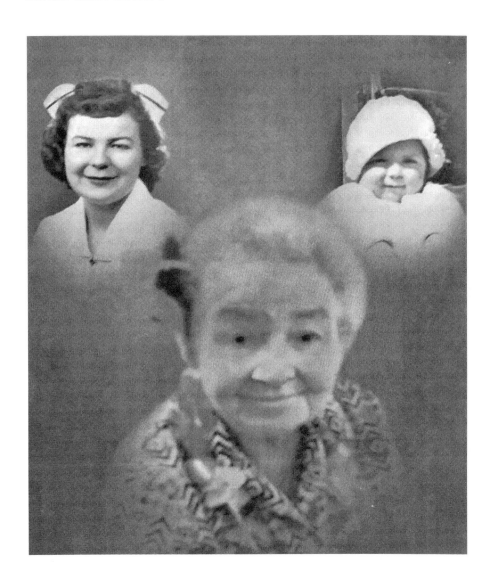

My father spent two years in the U. S. Army before I was born. He was in the Army from 1951 to 1953. Most of the time, he spent in Trieste, Italy fixing tanks.

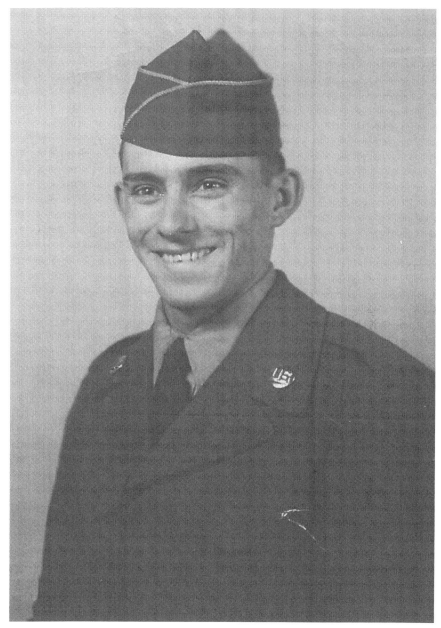

I was not very athletic as a child. I was good enough to be on the team, but not good enough to star on the team. I played Little League baseball, summer league park baseball, and I made the baseball team in junior high school. I never hit a home run. I did not play any other sports (basketball, football, or soccer).

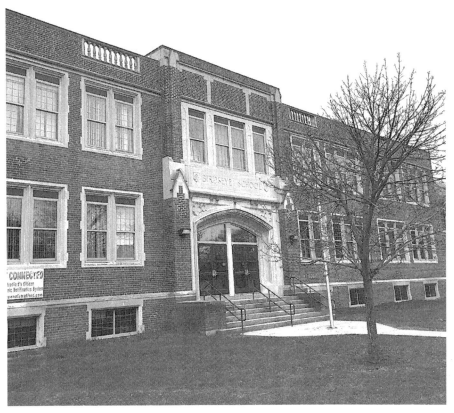

Dan's Elementary School

I was on a Saturday morning bowling league at around age 13. As mentioned earlier, I bowled in high school and received a high school varsity letter for bowling. We were required to have two physical education classes in college. I took bowling twice to meet that requirement.

When I was 15 years old, I had radio broadcasting training for several months at the Connecticut School of Broadcasting in Stratford, CT. I never used this training. Around the same time, I also took an "Evelyn Woods Speed Reading Dynamics" course. It was about six weeks long. I used what I learned a lot in my professional career.

My first job was at the Stratford Town Fair when I was 16 years old. I worked there for several years. I met Tereza (Terri) Marguy there, the love of my life. I was attracted to her beautiful green eyes, her dark hair, and her fun personality. She worked in the Stationary Department. I worked throughout the department store doing maintenance. Our first date was on April 30, 1972. We went bowling with another couple that worked at the Stratford Town Fair. Our second date, a week later, was to watch The Godfather in a movie theatre. We also went to the More's first anniversary party in Bridgeport, CT. (Tereza's sister Elena and her husband, Ronnie.) Our favorite song was "It's So Nice to Be with You" by Gallery.

I worked at the Stratford Town Fair until I took a job at Nichols Engineering in June 1973.

When I was an adult, I took karate lessons for three years (1984 to 1987) in Stratford, CT. When I moved to Pennsylvania, it took me two years to join another karate studio. I also took karate lessons there for three years (1989 to 1992).

I achieved the level of a blue belt, which was just below a black belt. At that point, I would assist the teacher in teaching class. Therefore, I was not learning anything new, and I did not feel I was prepared to take the black belt test. Consequently, I never became a black belt in karate.

Churches

I attended the following churches throughout my life.

Christ Episcopal Church, Stratford, CT, 1954-1973. Episcopal. This is the church I went to as a child before Jesus Christ saved me.

Stratford Baptist Church, Stratford, CT, 1973-1987. Baptist. This is the first church we went to as Bible-believing, born again, saved by grace Christians. My parents also started going to this church in 1973. Terri and I renewed our marriage vows there on our 25th Wedding Anniversary.

Country and Town Baptist Church, Mechanicsburg, PA, 1987-1992. Baptist. Brittany and Kelly had their baby dedications here. Jen and Karen had their wedding ceremonies here in 1995 and 2000, respectively.

Bible Baptist Church, Shiremanstown, PA, 1993-2002. Baptist. We were in the Dyson small group. Danielle graduated from Bible Baptist School. Brittany went to Bible Baptist School through 9th grade. Kelly went there through 7th grade. Because we are advocates of Christian schools, we started a scholarship fund at Bible Baptist School called the Kovlak Scholarship Fund. We have been supporting Christian schools for many years. This school is now part of the Christian School Association of Greater Harrisburg. (CSAGH)

Covenant Life Church, Gaithersburg, MD, 2002–2012. Sovereign Grace. Over the years, we were in the Pons Care Group, the Janson Care Group, and the Greer Care Group. We also served as assistant group leaders for the Alpha sessions for several years. I went on 2 one-week long mission trips to Juarez, Mexico, with Brittany in 2004 and with Kelly in 2006. Brittany and Kelly each graduated from Covenant Life Christian School. Brittany got married in Covenant Life Church in 2009.

Living Hope Church, Harrisburg, Middletown, PA, 2012 to present. Sovereign Grace. For several years, I was a collection counter every four weeks with Tom Shaheen. I also ran the Angel Tree Christmas program for the church for 2016, 2017, and 2018. We were in Gabe Krep's Community Group.

Brian Peters Jr., my oldest grandson, went to church with me while he was attending Messiah College. On the way, we would usually stop at Starbucks to pick up coffee and breakfast.

Daybreak Church, Mechanicsburg, PA, 2018 to present. Assembly of God. We did not officially become members, but we attend most of their small group meetings and events. Jen and Brian are members and also go to the small group meetings and events. Mark and Lu Shuey are our group leaders. We started going to church services in 2018.

Carlisle Reformed Presbyterian Church, Carlisle, PA, 2017 to present. Presbyterian (PCA). I am not a member of this church, but I go to most Sunday evening services. Living Hope Church and Daybreak Church do not have a Sunday Evening Service. I was introduced to this church when Dave Waterman, CBMC, invited me to the monthly Men's Bible Study breakfast around 2014. I still attend the breakfasts, when possible. During the 2020 pandemic, I participated in the services via live-stream from Florida.

Waypoint Church, Ponte Vedra, FL, 2020 to present, Presbyterian (PCA). I am not a member of this church. I attend here with the Boisvert family when I am in Florida. I also participate in the Wednesday Evening Men's Bible Study and the Friday morning Prayer Meeting on Zoom.

Charlie "Tremendous" Jones said that a donation to God's church was not "giving to God," but it was "returning to God." I like this saying. It is so true.

I have been blessed to go to the U.S. Banner of Truth conference almost every year, beginning in 2011. The conference is usually held in Elizabethtown, PA. The conference is 2½ days of excellent sermons each year.

Colleges

I went to college at the University of New Haven. I went there for four years from September 1972 through May 1976. I graduated with a degree in accounting.

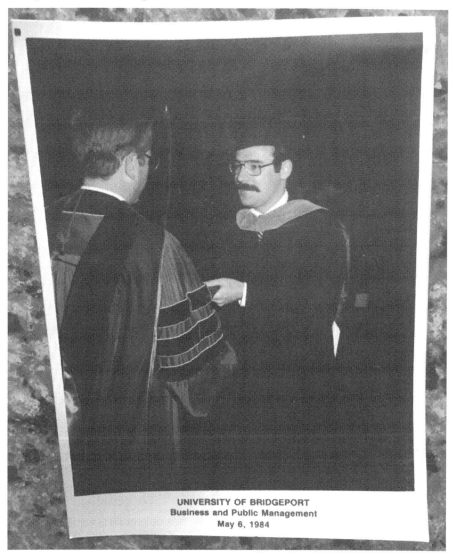

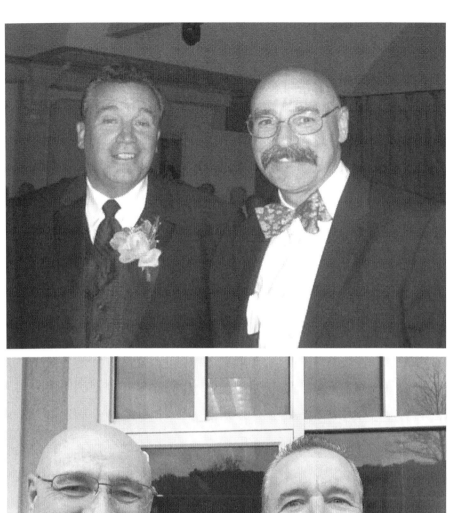
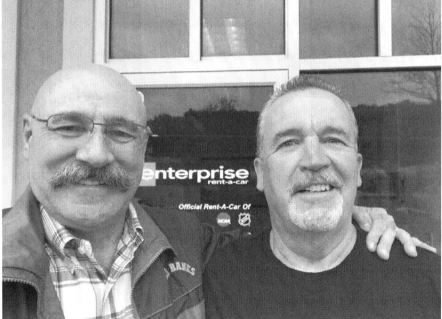

Dan & Fred

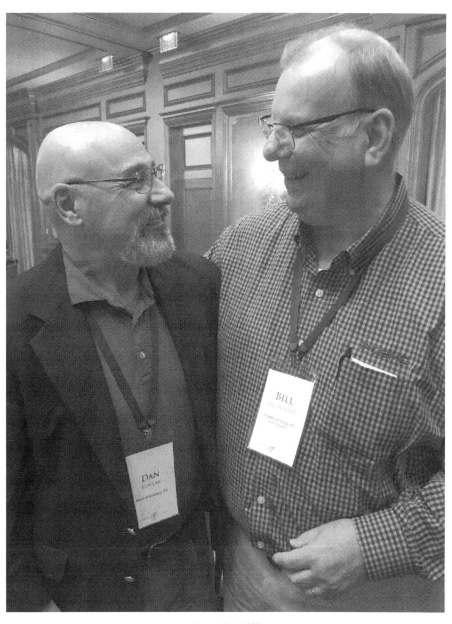

Dan & Bill

I went to every class and drove every day with Fred Vincent. We have been life-long friends.

He also majored in accounting. He joined a corporation upon graduation, and I joined a CPA firm, Peat, Marwick, Mitchell & Co. (Later It became KPMG.)

I had very good grades in college, averaging approximately 3.5 GPA. I also worked full time at Nichols Engineering while I went to college full-time. I was married for the last three years and had one child.

I would go to college from 8 AM until noon. Then I would come home, have lunch, and work at Nichols Engineering from 2 PM to 10 PM. My boss, John Kopchick, gave me flexible hours and also let me work on some Saturdays to make extra money. I worked in the machine shop at Nichols Engineering. I would come home and do homework until midnight and then sleep until morning and start all over again.

In 2019, I had dinner with Bill and Ginny McAvinney. Bill was the President of the Christian Business Men's Connection. While discussing how God has blessed us throughout our lives, we found out that Bill and I graduated from the University of New Haven on the exact same day in 1976. We had different majors, so we did not know each other then. Forty-three years later and 950 miles away from New Haven, we met each other because we are brothers in Christ!

I received my master's degree in business administration with a major in finance from the University of Bridgeport. I started my MBA after I had passed the CPA exam in 1979. I decided that the master's degree would give me a little extra in the business world. I took master's degree classes at night after work. I would attend classes two or three nights per week for several years. I received my master's degree in 1983.

Daily Routine

My morning routine has changed since I retired. When I worked, I got ready in less than an hour, took the train to DC in the morning, worked until about 6:30 PM. Then, I would return home.

Since I retired on September 30, 2012, I wake up at approximately 6:30 each morning. While I am making the bed, I listen to the Star-Spangled Banner on Alexa. (See chapter on Morning Routine.)

Because I have to be slower and more methodical because of my balance problem, it takes me about one hour and 15 minutes to get ready for the day.

I do devotions each day using the "Voices from the Past, Volumes 1 and 2" devotional books. Bill Geiger wrote a book on daily devotions (Personal Spiritual Growth). He attended our Daybreak Church small group meetings for six weeks to explain to us the importance of daily devotions.

I usually attend the Mechanicsburg CBMC weekly meeting at 6:30 AM on Mondays. Every two months, we have an evening board meeting for M28 Ministry (a Discipleship organization) on Zoom.

Some of the things that I do routinely are: I exercise 1/2 hour on the stationary recumbent bike. I also do exercises at home, with rubber exercise bands. When I arrived in Florida, I was exercising at the YMCA for two hours every other day. In Pennsylvania, I was doing water exercises, not swimming and not water aerobics, Monday, Wednesday, and Friday at a Physical Therapy water pool. Each day, I try to take a nap from approximately 1 to 3 PM or 2 to 4 PM.

On Tuesday nights, I usually attend Lions Club Zoom meetings with the Harrisburg Lions Club members. Before the coronavirus, we would have lunch meetings at the Harrisburg Hilton on the first and third Tuesdays of each month.

On Wednesday night, when I am in Florida, I usually have a Zoom meeting with the Waypoint Church Men's Bible Study group. On Friday morning at 8:00, I participate in the Zoom Prayer meeting of Waypoint Church.

On Sunday mornings, I try to live-stream the Black Rock Church service at 8:30. I live-stream the Carlisle Reformed Presbyterian Church service at 10:45 AM or The Palm Vista Church in Miami at 10:30 AM (This is the church that my oldest grandson, Brian Peters Jr., goes to.), or Waypoint Church at 10:30 AM.

At 6 PM, there is a live-streamed evening service at the Carlisle Reformed Presbyterian Church, which I usually attend. At almost every sermon I attend, I take copious notes. I have been doing this for several years. This helps me concentrate on the message and to absorb what I hear. The notes are also available for future review.

In between Zoom meetings, I continue to be active as the Treasurer of the Harrisburg Lions Club, work on jigsaw puzzles, play Sudoku, play Words with Friends, do "paperwork," and read audiobooks.

I usually listen to Fox News each day for 1 hour or so to stay current. I find them more credible than some of the other stations. To relax and not be too concerned about news events, I listen to Christian songs and oldies from the 1950s, 60s, and 70s. I have 2 Amazon playlists.

I prefer Old Time Gospels songs for my Christian songs playlist, but I have some more modern Christian songs and groups. The Gospel Song singers include Alan Jackson, Johnny Cash, Elvis Presley, The Inspirations, The Mormon Tabernacle Choir, The Wonder Kids, and Christian Gospel Choir. More modern Christian singing groups include Sovereign Grace Music.

I listen to 50s on 5, 60s on 6, and Fox News on Sirius XM radio. I also listen to Grace To You podcasts and other podcasts that have been recommended to me. I also communicate daily with my daughters using an app named "Marco Polo." This is like corresponding with text messages, but it uses video on the phone or tablet.

Egypt Trip

Brittany, Kelly, and I went on a trip to Egypt with Sherif Ettefa in 2007. Before we went to Egypt, we got an international cell phone from the phone company. (Later, you will understand its importance.)

Sherif was going there to visit his family because he was raised in Egypt. I knew Sherif from working with him in the Washington DC office of KPMG. We worked on several engagements together, and we became friends. Terri encouraged us to go with him. Terri did not like to fly and did not go.

We flew from Dulles airport in Virginia to Paris, France. After a short layover, we flew from Paris to Cairo. We slept in Cairo. Very early the next morning, we flew down to Aswan, where we started our riverboat cruise up the Nile River. While we were in Aswan, we saw the Aswan dam. That is a big tourist attraction.

On the cruise, we had dinner each night with a family from Australia. The family included a man, his wife, and her mother. Brittany and Kelly still keep in contact with them. The cruise ship was not very big since it was a riverboat. There were only about 200 people on the boat. The food was delicious. One night, on the cruise, we all got dressed up in Egyptian clothing. It was very amusing. It took several days of stopping at various temples and monuments to get to Cairo.

Once we were in Cairo, we crossed the river to go to Giza. While in Giza, we saw the pyramids. We did not go inside the pyramids. We thought it would be too claustrophobic.

We had camel rides for about 45 minutes and homemade bread cooked on an open hearth with some Bedouin Indians. Because the Indians were located about an hour from Giza, we were concerned about the safety of our ride out into the middle of the desert. We also went on a tour of a rug factory and a perfume factory. One of the Egyptian men offered to trade me several camels for Brittany. LOL.

We went to the Cairo Museum and saw a mummy exhibit. We visited Sharm El Sheik. It has a beautiful beach. Many worldwide diplomatic meetings are held there. We went to the Hard Rock Café while we were there.

After we spent several days in Giza and Sharm El Sheik, we took a taxi ride to Alexandria from Giza (several hours) to visit Sherif and his relatives. It was difficult getting to Alexandria because the driver did not speak any English, and we did not speak Arabic. We had to get Sherif's father on the phone to talk to the driver to arrive at the proper location. That was also very scary. Thank God for cell phones.

We stayed in a hotel in Alexandria for several days. We also saw the Alexandria library and a home for retarded children that Sherif's mother started. The library is one of the biggest libraries in the world.

After meeting with Sherif's family for several days, we went back to Cairo in a cab. The next day we flew from Cairo to Paris and then back to Dulles Airport in Virginia.

It was very hot in the summer in Egypt. It was around 100°. The water in the Mediterranean Sea was a beautiful blue/green color. I also had Turkish coffee there, which was very strong.

Sherif's father made all of the arrangements for the trip. I simply sent him a check for the entire cost. His father is a retired CPA in Egypt. Many thanks to him, Sherif, and the rest of the family for the lifetime memories we made in Egypt.

Family
Family Tree

When I was born, I had two grandfathers and two grandmothers. By the time I was 8, both grandfathers and one grandmother died. Therefore, I only knew the one surviving grandmother, Alice Rosamond Begelspiker Sterbinsky (1897 to 1976). She died when I was 21 years old.

She was my mother's mother. She lived in Bridgeport, Connecticut. She was 80 years old when she died. She worked in American Fabrics Lace factory her entire adult life until she was 65. She had two sisters that I also knew: Aunt Minnie and Aunt Margaret.

They were my mother's aunts. My mother had one brother and one sister. (Frank, 1922 to 1999, and Ethel, 1918 to 1968). Frank had six children: four girls and two boys. Ethel had five sons. My mother's name was Hilma Sterbinsky Kovlak. She lived from 1929 until 2011.

My father had three brothers and one sister. (Joseph - 1910 to 1970, Leonard - 1924 to 2002, Donald - 1939 to 2010, and Helen -1912 to 1988). My father's name was Vincent Martin Kovlak Sr. He lived from 1930 until 2006. My father's mother had 13 children from 1910 until 1939. However, only five of those children lived.

I did not know three of my grandparents: my father's mother and father, Francis Tribble (1891 to 1963), and Daniel Joseph Kovlak (1889 to 1959). My other grandfather, whom I did not know, was Frank Arthur Sterbinsky (1889 to 1961).

My first name, Daniel, was my father's father's first name. My middle name came from my father's boss's first name (my father's friend and mentor). His name was Leslie Poinelli. He went by the name Les.

Joe had no children. Leonard had four children: three girls and one boy. Helen had no children, and Donald had no children.

My father's uncle's name was Henry Tribble (1907 to 1998). He was my grandmother's brother. He was a very nice guy. He was always jovial. His wife's name was Anna. She had severe arthritis until she died. They had no children. They lived in Shelton, CT.

My great grandparents were:

John Sterbinsky (1859 to 1900)

Regina Rosalia Krakovsky (1864 to 1929)

John Begelspiker (1851 to 1910)

Mary Miller (1856 to 1908)

Daniel Joseph Kovlak (Kovalyak) (1865 to 1942)

Anne Helen Porvaznik (1866 to 1919)

Martin Tribble (Tryba) (1869 to 1939)

Sophia Konieczny (1870 to 1945)

Family Physical Stature and Eye Colors

I am 5'9" and weigh about 180 lbs. (brown eyes). My mother was 5'0" and weighed about 130 lbs. (green eyes). My father was 5'5" and weighed about 160 lbs. (brown eyes).

My grandparents were:

Mother's mother 4'11", 180 lbs. (brown eyes)

Mother's father, 5'2", 150 lbs. (brown eyes)

Father's mother, 5'5", 175 lbs. (blue eyes)

Father's father, 6'0', 210 lbs. (brown eyes)

My father's brothers and sister were:

Joe, 6'3", 200 lbs. (blue eyes)

Leonard, 6'2", 200 lbs. (blue eyes)

Donny, 5'10", 180 lbs. (blue eyes)

Helen, 5'4", 175 lbs. (blue eyes)

The Kovlak name will disappear from this branch of the Kovlak family after this generation. My grandfather Daniel Joseph Kovlak had four sons to carry on the name. Of his four sons, the oldest and youngest had no children (Joe and Donny). Leonard had one son, and Vinny (my father) had two sons. Leonard's son had no children. Of the two sons that Vinny had (my brother and me), I had five girls and no boys; my brother had four girls and one boy. His son has no children. Therefore, the Kovlak name will be gone soon.

Immediate Family

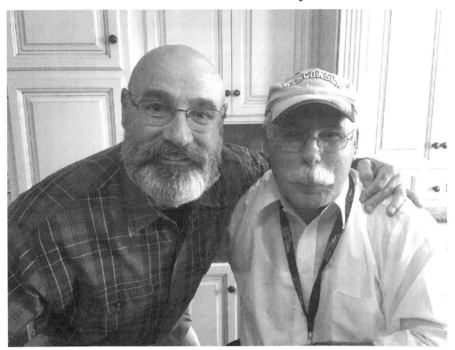

Danny & Vinny

Tereza (Terri) and I have five daughters, and currently, 18 grandchildren. I love my wife, daughters, and every one of my grandchildren. They are all a true blessing from God.

Of the 18 grandchildren, we have seven boys and eleven girls.

Jennifer – three boys and two girls

Karen – one boy and one girl

Danielle – one boy and two girls

Brittany – two boys and two girls

Kelly – four girls.

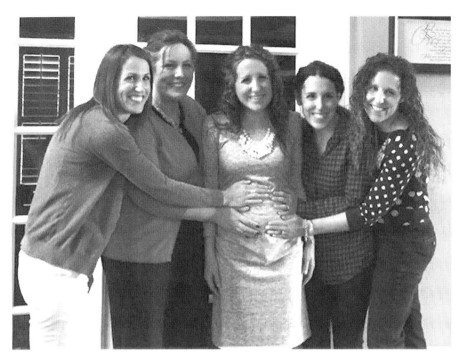

5 Daughters

Each of our daughters has graduated from college with majors in the following areas: Jennifer – Elementary Ed – Liberty University; Karen – Nursing – Harrisburg Area Community College; Danielle – Elementary Ed – Baptist Bible College and East Stroudsburg University; Brittany – Accounting – University of Maryland; and Kelly – Nursing – Liberty University and Penn State University at Hershey Medical Center.

They are all married.

I enjoyed teaching each of the girls how to drive a car in preparation for their drivers' tests. After we were married, I also taught Terri how to drive a stick shift car. We had a 1963 stick shift car at the time. I taught her this on a hilly area near our house; we called "Suicide Hill." I never drove a motorcycle in my life. My parents thought they were too dangerous.

Although they are not supposed to be hereditary, two of our daughters had two different types of hemangiomas as babies.

When Karen and Danielle were in high school, they were cheerleaders for football and wrestling. We went to high school wrestling matches for several years. This gave us a great appreciation for the sport of wrestling as well as interest in Mixed Martial Arts years later.

One tradition that we started was "back to school shopping" with the girls. Each year, they would get a list of items that they would need for the school year. Before school started, we would make "back to school" shopping a traditional event that we looked forward to each year.

As parents, we learned that when two children share a food or dessert, one person cuts, and the other chooses their piece first. That way, the cutter is sure to cut evenly.

I also learned that "there is no time like the present time," so don't procrastinate.

For some years, around Christmas, we have sent out our Kovlak Family, "Year in Review," to friends and relatives. This is a good way of documenting things that our family did during the year. Also, a day or two before New Year's Eve, when most of the girls and their families are at our house to celebrate New Year's Eve with us, we have started a tradition of "Breakfast with Pops." All of the girls go out to breakfast with me, and we enjoy each other's company.

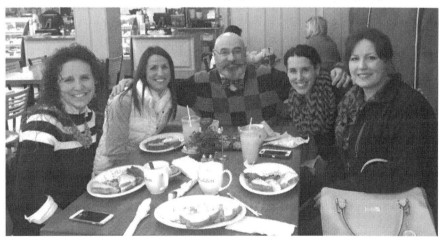

Breakfast with Pops

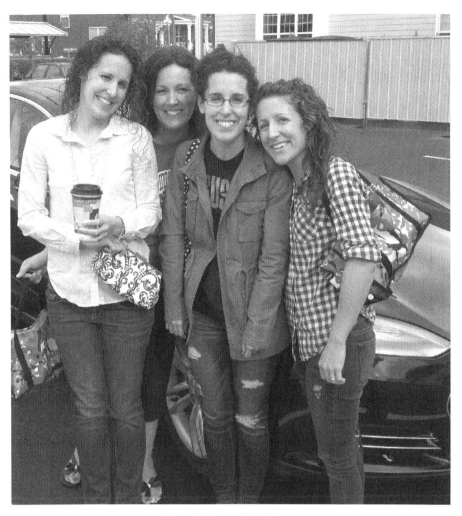

Breakfast with Pops

One tradition that Terri started was the "12 days of Christmas" Tradition. For each of the 12 days that lead up to Christmas Day, she would give each of the girls a small gift. I buy for Terri, and she buys for me. This tradition has been carried down to the next generation.

Another tradition that Terri started was to have a Christian sign or symbol in each room of our house to be a constant reminder of God's presence. The one I like the most is the sign that we have in our kitchen that says,"'I saw that!' God"

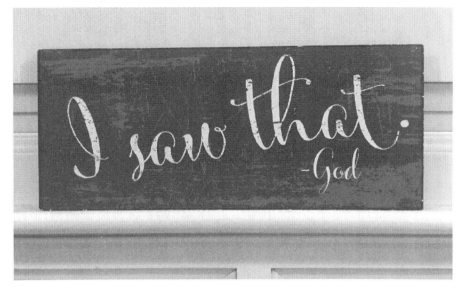

Famous People

Terri and I have met the following famous people.

Bob and Libby Dole, former United States Senators. Bob was also a candidate for President in 1996. We met them at the PICPA Dinner in Pittsburgh around 2000.

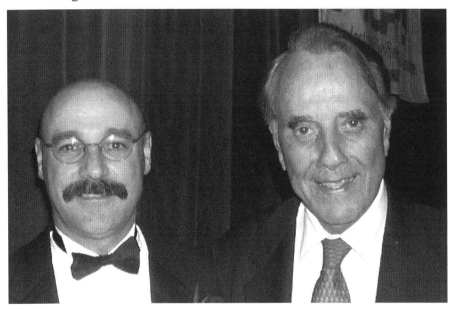

Dan & Bob Dole

Newt Gingrich. Former Speaker of the House of Representatives. We met him at one of the central Pennsylvania political dinners around 1990.

G. Gordon Liddy. He worked for President Nixon and went to jail in the Watergate scandal. We met him at our niece's confirmation ceremony in Virginia. His granddaughter was also getting confirmed. That was around the year 2000.

Jim Bunning. He pitched a perfect game for the Philadelphia Phillies in 1964. He later became a United States Senator from Kentucky. We met him at a fund-raising picnic around 1990.

Alan Greenspan. He was the Federal Reserve Board (FRB) Chairman from 1987 to 2006. Because the FRB was one of my clients, I presented the financial statements to him at one of their board meetings around 2005.

Phil Mickelson. Professional golfer. We met him at the KPMG Partners Meeting in Orlando in 2012. He wears the KPMG hat in all of his golf tournaments.

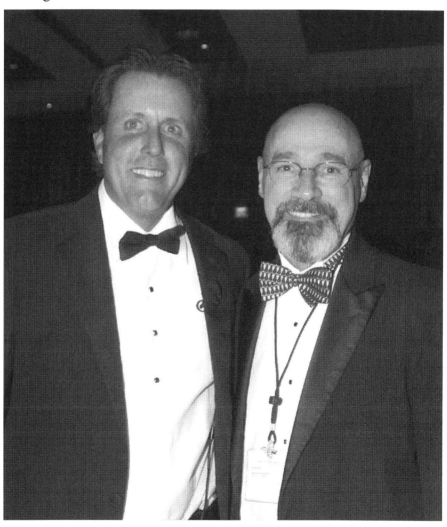

Phil Michelson & Dan

Mark Whitacre. He had a book written and a movie made about his life titled "The Informant." We met him around 2014 through CBMC. He and his wife Ginger are very close friends now. He is also a great Christian brother.

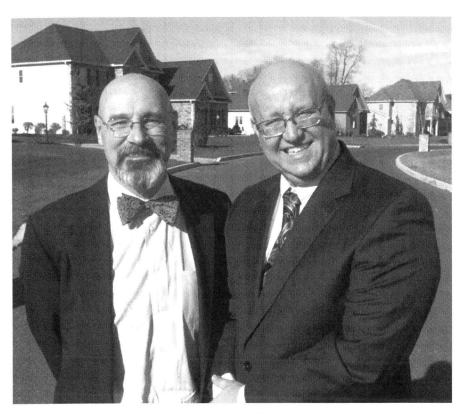

Dan & Mark Whitacre

Favorite Books

I started listening to audiobooks at age 55. One of the nice things about them is you can listen to them as you are driving. You can also back them up or go forward as much as you want. There are a tremendous number of books available, although not all books come in an audio format. I buy an annual number of credits from Audible and use them throughout the year. There are various other suppliers of audiobooks. I also buy Kindle books, which, in many cases, have an audio function.

Goodreads is an excellent app for readers. You can keep track of the books you have read, the dates that you read them, your rating of the book, your review of the book, and others' ratings and reviews.

Christian books

Voices from the Past (Volume 1 and Volume 2) by Richard Rushing
ESV Study Bible
Operation Timothy books by CBMC
Systematic Theology and Bible Doctrine by Wayne Grudem
The Attributes of God by Arthur Pink

Secular books

The Count of Monte Cristo

Uncle Tom's Cabin

The Devil in the White City

Letitia Baldwin's New Complete Guide to Executive Manners (an essential book for business people)

Life is Tremendous (Charlie Jones also had three excellent songs sung by Don Wooten: Life is Tremendous, Read Books, and Confidence. The words in these songs are tremendous, and the tunes are very catchy.)

The Ultimate Gift

Gilead

Funny Things

Songs

In the 1960s and 1970s, there were some very creative and funny songs. Some of them are listed below.

A Boy Named Sue,

One Piece at a Time,

Camp Grenada,

My Mother-in-law,

Pick an Ugly Woman to be Your Wife,

Henry the 8th,

Beep, Beep,

King of the Road,

You Talk Too Much.

"We Are Family", by Sister Sledge, is a song that our daughters dance to at weddings and other festive events. It describes nicely the relationships that our five daughters have. Praise God.

Stories

This is the longest chapter in this book. After many years of a blessed life, I have many funny stories to tell. I hope you get enjoyment from these stories.

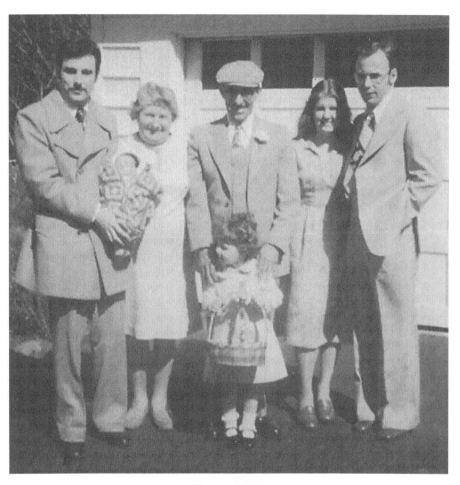

Easter 1977

Easter

For years, my aunt made a traditional Easter breakfast at about ten AM Easter Sunday each year. She would have all the food blessed at the church the day before. She would also have several very time consuming, handmade items for breakfast. She put a a lot of time and effort into the traditional breakfast.

After he graduated from college, my brother became a pastor. One of his responsibilities was to perform the church service on Easter Sunday. His service was approximately the same time as the traditional breakfast. Therefore, he could not attend the breakfast that began at 10 AM.

Ironically, my aunt said, "It is a shame that Vinny has to ruin Easter by going to church." LOL.

Ted Williams Tunnel Dedication

Ted Williams was one of the best baseball players in baseball history. He played for the Boston Red Sox. Boston built a tunnel underneath the city, which is about 2 miles long. They named this tunnel the Ted Williams Tunnel. At the dedication ceremony, the person sitting next to Ted Williams wanted to make conversation.

Knowing that the average baseball player makes well over $1 million a year, this person asked Ted Williams, being one of the best players in baseball history, how much money he thought he would make if he played baseball today.

Ted Williams said, "Oh, maybe about $1 million." The other person said, "Only $1 million? Why so little when the average person is making several million dollars per year?"

Ted Williams responded that "You have to realize that I am almost 80 years old." LOL.

Mobster Story

A mobster boss's only brother died. The mobster boss went to the priest who was going to perform the service. The mobster boss told the priest, although his brother had committed serious crimes, he would like the priest to say that his brother was a saint.

The mobster boss assured the priest that he would give the church a significant contribution after saying this. The priest thought about this for a while, and then he told the mobster boss that he would do it.

During the service, the priest said that the mobster boss's brother "was a thief, a scoundrel, a liar, and a murderer, but he was a saint compared to his brother." LOL.

Dental Patient

An elderly lady went to a dentist for the first time. While she was in the waiting room, she saw that the diploma on the wall indicated that the dentist went to the same high school and they graduated together.

After he performed her dental services, she said to him, "I think you and I were in the same high school class together."

He said to her, "What did you teach?" Obviously, he thought she looked much older than him. LOL.

Taco Bell Story

One day Tony Marguy (my father-in-law, who was around 90 years old at the time) and I were going to drive from Gaithersburg, Maryland to Mechanicsburg, Pennsylvania. Before the trip, we decided to pick up Taco Bell food for dinner in the car.

I asked him if he wanted a quesadilla. He laughed. I asked him again if he wanted a quesadilla. He laughed again. Finally, I ordered him a quesadilla. When Taco Bell gave it to me, I gave it to him.

He said, "What is this?" I said, "It is a quesadilla."

He started laughing and said that he thought I was ordering him a case of beer. LOL.

Expert Speaker

An expert speaker on technical issues was with his driver one day. The driver said that "I have heard your speech so many times, I could give it myself." The expert speaker said, "OK, I will stand in the back of the room in the audience and watch you."

The driver performed the speech flawlessly with the expert in the back of the room. During the question and answer session, a question came up that the speaker, the driver, could not answer.

Therefore, he said to the audience, "That question is so simple, I think I'll give it to my car driver to answer." LOL.

Small Gift

A child got a money gift for his birthday from a relative. The child thanked the relative for the gift by saying, "Thank you for the small gift."

The gift-giver was so annoyed that he said he would never give that person a birthday gift again. LOL.

Discolored Plant

From 2005 to 2010, my mother owned a townhouse in Shiremanstown, PA. The Peters family (my daughter and her family) had another townhouse. Terri and I had a third townhouse that we would stay in on weekends when we visited my father, who was in a nursing home. (All three townhouses were in the same section of the Shiremanstown townhouses.) While my mother was there, I took responsibility for the maintenance of her townhouse.

One day, I saw a huge weed growing in her yew bushes in front of the house. I tried to pull the weed out, but it was like a tree trunk growing in the middle of the yew bush.

Therefore, I cut it down as low as the yew bush and sprayed weed killer on it. The next week, when I came back to the townhouse, the weed was dead, but so was the yew bush's center portion. It was brown, and the rest of the yew was dark green.

Rather than digging up the yew bushes and putting in new yew bushes, I decided to take a green branch from the yew bush to the Home Depot.

I purchased a can of spray paint with the color that was most like the green branch. I came back and sprayed the yew's dead branches with green spray paint so it would look like the rest of the bush. Eventually, the new branches grew in.

I saved myself a lot of work and money by not digging up the yews and planting new ones.

Dr. Sarosi

When I was in college in New Haven, CT, one of my professors was a professor of economics named Dr. Sarosi.

Dr. Sarosi was about 80 years old. He was single, born in Hungary, brought up in Texas, and lived permanently in a hotel room in downtown New Haven. He had a Hungarian accent with a Texas drawl!

He wore the same suit every day. It was a brown herringbone, wool suit with a vest. He was very short and skinny.

Examples of what he said follow:

If you were a few minutes late for class, he would say: "Vere have you beeannnnnnn boysssss? I have bean vating for you?"

If you wore jeans that day, he would say:

"Answer my question, you dunjereened young maan."

If you had a mustache, he would call you a "mustahshioed young maan."

One day, when we had a break in our class, we talked with another student who drove his car to the university. Our fellow student told us the following story about the professor. One day, the student knew the professor was finished with his classes for the day and was going home. So he asked the professor if he could give him a ride home to downtown New Haven. The professor agreed, so they got into the car.

They were only driving about 2 miles to downtown New Haven, Connecticut, where Dr. Sarosi lived in the hotel. As they were driving in the car, there was a traffic jam. The person in the car behind started beeping his horn and continued beeping his horn.

Finally, the student said, out loud, "Where do you want me to go, YOU JERK?"

The professor thought he was talking to him. In a matter of fact manner, the professor said, "You can drop me off at the drugstore."

The student was actually talking out loud in his car to the person honking the horn behind them. But, the professor thought he was talking to him. LOL.

Washington DC Cab Ride

When I worked at KPMG in Washington, DC, one of my clients was the Department of Treasury. Each federal agency was required to issue its audited financial statements by November 15 of each year.

As a result, we would work very long hours from the middle of October until the middle of November to complete the audits on time.

I would take the metro system to work and take it home. At that time, the latest Metro train was midnight.

One night, I got to the Metro at 11:30 PM. The sign at the Metro said they had operational problems, and the Metro would not be running the last train to Maryland, where I was going.

Because there were some people that wanted to go to Maryland, and there was no Metro going there, this man asked me if I would like to take a cab with him.

I did not know him, but I said, "yes." He also found a lady who was also going to Maryland. The three of us could split the cab fare.

As we were in the cab, each of us talked about our jobs and our backgrounds. There are thousands of universities all over the world. The three of us were working in DC at the time. The three of us met randomly.

During our conversation, we found that each of us were graduates of colleges in New Haven, CT! I was a graduate of the University of New Haven, the man was a graduate of Yale University, and the lady was a graduate of Southern Connecticut State College.

It is amazing that, of the number of people that work in Washington DC, three people getting in a cab randomly would have all gone to colleges in the same city 300 miles away!

The Apostle Paul

Recently I heard a sermon from Pastor John MacArthur. The sermon was about the book of Acts. He said that the Apostle Paul was significant in spreading the gospel, as documented in the book of Acts.

The Apostle Paul made three missionary journeys to numerous cities to spread the gospel over several decades. Ultimately, he went to Rome to be tried, told the Romans about the gospel, and was executed.

Dr. MacArthur indicated that Paul was so diligent about spreading the gospel throughout the world; if Paul hadn't been executed, he might have discovered America!

I thought this was amusing, and I also thought this was true.

Bond's Dock

When I was around 13 years old, after doing my paper route in Stratford, CT, which included about 30 newspaper deliveries, the paper route ended in an area called Bond's Dock, near the Stratford Shakespearean Theater.

Bond's Dock was where people would launch their boats into the Housatonic River with their trailers. People would also fish at Bond's Dock. It was said that it was dangerous to swim there because of undercurrents.

My brother heard that a bicycle would float if it has air in the tires. We wanted to test out this theory. Therefore, my brother rode my bike off of Bond's Dock into the Housatonic River.

Unfortunately, the bike did not float. It went to the bottom of the river! My brother was able to escape unharmed. My brother, my friends, and I were all bewildered. Fortunately, there was a boat repair facility next to Bond's Dock. They lent us a rope and a grappling hook to fish the bike out of the river.

After an hour or so, we were able to fish the bike out of the water. The water was approximately 15 feet deep. We were all surprised that we were able to get the bike back. This situation has led to lifelong memories.

The Book of Revelation

A well-to-do businessman went to get his shoes shined by a shoeshine boy. The businessman saw that the shoeshine boy had a book that he was reading. He asked the shoeshine boy what he was reading. He responded that he was reading the Bible.

He then asked what book of the Bible he was reading. The response was the book of Revelation. Knowing that this book is very prophetic and, at times, hard to understand, the businessman condescendingly asked what this complicated book meant to the shoeshine boy.

His response was, "Jesus Wins."

That is a beautiful response. It is so simple and so true.

Highway Ride

One day, an elderly man (around 90 years old) was driving down a superhighway rapidly. His wife called him to tell him to be careful on that specific highway because she heard on the radio that someone was on that same highway driving in the wrong direction.

His response to her was, "That's not bad, the road that I am on, ALL of the other drivers are driving in the wrong direction!"

Dinner Prayer

A little boy asked his friend if he prayed before dinner. His response was, "No, my Mom is a good cook."

Clients

I tell people that I was with the same CPA firm for over 35 years. I also tell them that in the CPA profession, auditor turnover is about 70% because, quite often, our clients like their auditor, offers him/her a job, and then the auditor leaves the firm.

Then I tell people that I was with the same firm for a long time because none of my clients liked me! LOL

Glass of Water

A little boy went to bed at bedtime. After a few minutes, he called from the top of the stairs and said to his Dad that he wanted some water. His Dad said, "No, now go to bed." The boy asked his father again for a glass of water. The father said, "No," again. The boy asked his Dad for a third time for a glass of water. This time his father said, "No, and if you ask again, I will come up there and discipline you."

The boy said, "When you come up to discipline me, can you bring me a glass of water?" LOL

The Idiot Book

During an Outer Banks vacation, one of my daughters was reading the book, The Idiot, by Theodore Dostoyevsky. It was a thick book. One of my grandsons wanted to know what book she was reading. She answered him by saying, "I am reading the book The Idiot, and right now, I'm reading the chapter about you!" LOL.

Post Card

When I was around 12 years old, one of my my friends went on a vacation. In his travels, he visited a historic cemetery. As a joke, he sent me a postcard with a picture of the cemetery. He wrote on the postcard, "I wish you were here." with an arrow pointing to one of the graves. I thought that was very funny and creative.

Egg Sandwiches

When I worked at Nichols Engineering, I had a wonderful boss. Sometimes, he would let me work Saturday morning so I could earn a little extra money. He was very generous. On Saturdays, he would offer to buy us egg sandwiches for breakfast. At that time, I did not like egg sandwiches. He would go around to each employee and ask them if he could buy them an egg sandwich. When he came to me, I would politely say, "no, thank you." He was very persistent and asked several times. Each time, I politely said, "No." Finally, I said, "OK." He then said to me, "DON'T YOU EVER SAY 'NO.'" LOL.

Rice

One day, when one of my daughters was in high school, she went out to dinner with her friends. One of her friends ate some very delicious rice. She commented on how good the rice was and said, "I wonder what kind of rice this is?" Another friend said that they thought it was Condoleezza Rice. The response was, "That sure is good rice!"

(The funny part of the story is that Condoleezza Rice was the name of the Attorney General of the United States at the time. The person answering knew that, but the person enjoying the rice did not know that.) LOL.

White Belt

Early in my career, I was attending a meeting of the National Association of Accountants. In that meeting, our speaker was talking about improving management techniques. He told this story, which I will remember for the rest of my life.

He said that a management position opened up where he worked. All of the employees knew that a particular person should be promoted to that position. However, someone else was promoted to that position.

When management was asked why the person who deserved the position did not get it, management explained that the person that was passed over wore a white belt. (White belts were considered unprofessional at that time.) The other person asked the manager if anyone told that person that he should not wear a white belt to work. Management's response was, "We could not tell him not to wear a white belt because we did not want to hurt his feelings."

This shows that proper counseling is required for all positions. The counseling should be honest and confidential.

Car Trip

One time the Rauch Family came from CT to PA to visit us. They had three children. When they arrived, I noticed a $20 bill clipped to the visor. I asked why it was there. Bob told me that it was a constant reminder to the kids to behave during the car ride. He told them, at the beginning of the trip, that if they behaved in the car during the journey, they would get the money at the end of the long trip. I thought that was a great idea.

Tesla Onesie

Tesla is an electric car. Therefore, it has no emissions. Like most prominent companies, Tesla has items with their name, logo, or slogan on various items for sale. An example is a coffee mug.

At one point in time, Tesla had available for sale a babies' onesie that had printed on the front "no emissions." I thought that was a very creative way of using the term "emissions."

Assurance of Salvation

When I was a relatively new Christian and my brother was a young Pastor, he and I went door-to-door witnessing about Jesus. We went to a house nearby and knocked on the door. This lady answered the door. My brother asked her if she "had the assurance of salvation."

We could tell by the lady's accent that English was her second language. Her reply was: "I have plenty of INSURANCE." and slammed the door.

She thought we were door to door INSURANCE salesmen! (See the chapter on "Salvation.")

Yale University

Two young men were graduating from Yale University. They were at their commencement ceremony. The commencement speaker was an alumnus of Yale University. He was about 80 years old.

In his commencement speech, he began by saying Y stands for youth, and he described how important his education at Yale helped him during his youth. He talked about his youth for one hour.

He next talked about the A in Yale, which stood for academics. He described how vital the academics were at Yale, which helped him throughout his life. He went another hour on the letter A.

Then he got to the letter L, which stood for lifelong learning. He explained how this learning process helped him throughout his life. He spent one hour talking about lifelong learning.

Finally, he came to the letter E, which stood for education, and he described how the education he received at YALE was a lifetime benefit. He talked about that for one hour.

After four hours, he finished his speech.

After the commencement speech, one of the graduates asked the other one, "What did you think of the speech?" The other student said to him, "I sure am glad that we didn't go to the Massachusetts Institute of Technology." LOL.

Pops

When I am in Ponte Vedra, FL, sometimes I go to the dry cleaners. The first time I went there, there was a lady at the counter that was around my age. Her husband was there also.

As I was chatting with them, I learned that they have five daughters and no sons. I told them that we also have five daughters and no sons. I later asked what the grandchildren called their grandfather. They said, "Pops." I said that is what my grandchildren call me. I asked them what their grandchildren call their grandmother. They said, "Granny." I said that is what our grandchildren call their grandmother!

What are the chances that we would have so much in common with complete strangers?

Air Vent

A friend of mine moved into a house. He had the living room painted before he moved in. It was a huge room, about 40 feet long. Shortly after moving in, one of the upstairs bathrooms had a leak that stained the living room ceiling. The stain, about six inches in diameter, was quite visible on the newly painted white ceiling. Rather than have the entire ceiling repainted, he cut a hole in the ceiling where the stain was and put an air vent there. The air vent did not have any functional purpose, but it looked like it belonged there. He did not have to repaint the entire ceiling. I thought this was an ingenious idea!

Videos

Most of these videos you can get on YouTube.

Chevy Chase Videos
Stonehenge
Roundabout in London

Abbott and Costello Videos
Who's on First?
We Want Candy!

Other Videos
Little boy, who gets "Books for Christmas?"
Alan Iverson saying, "Practice?"
Barney's Clothing Store advertisement from the 1960s of little kids in New York City: Barney tells Mayor LaGuardia, Louis Armstrong, and Babe Ruth, "Everyone Needs Clothes."
Father Guido Sarducci explains the "5 Minute Degree."
In the TV show Taxi, when Jim is taking his driver's test.
In the Godfather movie, they say, "Who Pauly? You won't be seeing him no more."
Also, in the Godfather movie, they say, "Leave the gun, take the cannolis."
On Saturday Night Live, Linda Richmond says, "I am all verklempt."
On Saturday Night Live, Roseanne Roseannadanna says, "It's always somethin!" at the end of many of her situations.
Best Wife Ever - Blind Guy on a Motorbike
Don't Call Me Shirley! - Airplane Movie.
Amazon Echo Silver - SNL
I also like The Inspirations song, "I'm a Winner Either Way."

Gadgets

I love using gadgets. My latest gadget is a Rollator, which is a walker with wheels.

I also use Alexa quite a bit, which is an electronic personal assistant.

I also have an electric car. I did not get an electric car because I am concerned about saving the environment. I got it because it is a unique gadget at this time. I think, in the future, all cars and trucks will be electric. My car also has "Autopilot," which steers the vehicle (if there are lines in the road), and it also controls its speed. I also believe, in the not too distant future, all cars will fully drive themselves, and they will be much safer than the vehicles that we have now.

I like to listen to electronic audiobooks.

We also have a robotic vacuum cleaner.

The girls gave me an Apple Watch for Christmas. It does numerous things like a smartphone. But, if you fall, the watch will ask you if you need help. If you do not answer, it will automatically send help.

Governmental Accounting Standards Board (GASB)

The GASB was a newly created organization in 1984. It is the sister organization to the Financial Accounting Standards Board (FASB). The parent of both of those organizations is the Financial Accounting Foundation (FAF).

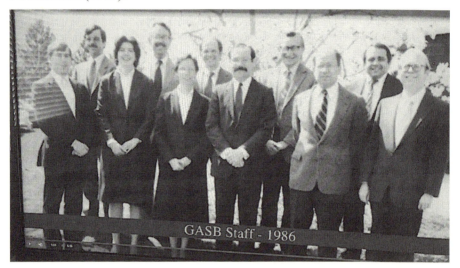

GASB Staff 1986

Jack Miller, KPMG's Vice Chairman - Government, asked me if I was interested in joining the GASB as its first Practice Fellow. That meant that I was an official employee of the GASB but was guaranteed a position with KPMG after two years. I worked at the GASB from September 1, 1984 to August 31, 1986. At that time, the GASB was located in Stamford, CT. I lived in Stratford, CT. My commute was approximately 25 miles one way. I went to the same location every day, unlike public accounting (auditing), where you go to the client's site almost every day.

I interviewed and was hired by the Vice Chairman of the GASB, Marty Ives. Marty was my boss for two years. The Chairman was Jim Antonio. They were both delightful to work with. The other staff at the GASB were also delightful to work with.

Before forming the GASB, accounting standards for the states and local governments were set by the National Committee on Governmental Accounting (NCGA). That was a volunteer organization with no paid staff.

When I was at the GASB, it was much more collegial than a CPA firm. In other words, there was a lot of research, discussion, and writing. Since the GASB was a newly formed organization for state and local governmental accounting, it affected almost every type of government throughout the country. Many people were interested in what we were doing. Therefore, the GASB employees were invited to speak to various government organizations throughout the country. I enjoyed speaking to others about the background, history, and progress that GASB was making.

I also made presentations to the five-member board monthly. In the 24 months that I worked at GASB, I made presentations to the board approximately 21 times. This was a great experience for me to interact, on current topics, with people that had much more experience than I did.

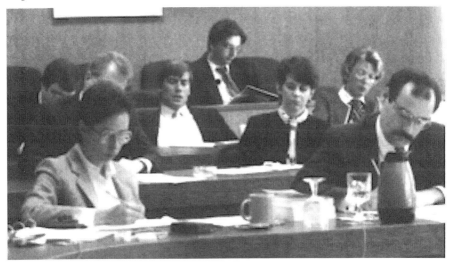

GASB Board Meeting

The final products that I worked on while I was there for two years was an Exposure Draft on the Measurement Focus/Basis of Accounting and a statement on Accounting and Reporting for

Investments, including Repurchase Agreements. The latter project dealt with a current issue in governments at that time. We hoped that better financial reporting for repurchase agreements would help governments avoid losing money by investing in repurchase agreements and other risky investment vehicles.

One day, while having a review of my draft document by one of the board members, he told me a story about business writing, which I will never forget.

He told me the story about a young man carrying a sign that said: "fresh fish for sale today." Someone came up to the young man and said, "fresh fish for sale today?" We know it is for sale today; take the word "today" off your sign. So, he did.

Then he walked around with the sign that said: "fresh fish for sale." The next person saw him and said, "fresh fish for sale?" We know the fish is fresh; otherwise, you would not be selling it. Then he crossed off the word "fresh" on his sign.

Now he was walking around with a sign that said: "fish for sale." As he walked around, another person came up to him and said, "fish for sale?" Why do you need the words "for sale"? We know if you have fish, it is for sale, so he took the words "for sale" off of his sign. Now his sign simply said, "fish."

The next person that looked at the sign said to him, "Why do you have a sign that says 'fish'"? "We know you have fish; we can smell it!"

The purpose of the story is to convey that when we have an idea, we should convey that idea in as few words as possible in business.

At GASB, we would go out every Friday for pizza. This was when I was introduced to pizza with onions and green peppers on it. This is still one of my favorites, and it is a favorite for some of my daughters too!

In 2009, GASB had a 25 Year Reunion. I went to that in Norwalk, CT. It was fantastic to reunite with many old friends. They also had a 30 Year Reunion in 2014. Unfortunately, I was unable to attend. However, GASB has a great recap of it on their website.

Golf

I started playing golf at age 21. I never became a very good golfer regardless of the number of lessons that I took, the equipment I bought, or practice. I believe that you should learn golf as a child. Then it will become easier for you.

However, even though I was not a very good golfer, I made many friends playing golf. One of my best friends and KPMG Partner was John Azzariti. I played golf with him several times in his member-guest tournament at the Ridgewood Country Club in Danbury, CT.

We joined Carlisle Country Club, as a family, on October 1, 1988. I made some friends there, including Paul Hertzler, my partner in many tournaments.

I joined the Carlisle Country Club Tuesday Night League in order to meet other people. Since the matches were set up by golf score handicaps and mine was so high, I got matched with most of the guys that were in their 80's (age, not score). LOL. I also became a board member.

Terri and I participated in their bowling league for several years.

Two of our daughters had their wedding receptions at the Carlisle Country Club. Terri and I also celebrated our 60th birthdays there, with many family members attending.

Hobbies

Now that I'm retired, I have more time for hobbies. I make jigsaw puzzles, exercise, play Words with Friends and Suduko, read (mostly audiobooks), pay bills, function as the Treasurer of the Harrisburg Lions Club, and do other paperwork.

I don't watch much TV. When I do, it is usually news or sports: professional football or college football, or MMA fighting. I do not watch basketball games or baseball games on TV. I do not play video games.

I have learned that the manufacturer of a jigsaw puzzle makes a big difference. I usually like 1000 pieces. However, some of the less expensive puzzles don't fit together tightly. When you put one piece in, six other pieces come out. Therefore, I would rather pay for a quality puzzle. I just started gluing my puzzles together. I think I will give them away as gifts as a remembrance of me. (My father did this with Christmas ornaments. However, he was much better at handiwork than me.)

I read a lot of books. Some of the books I have read are: The Bible, The Count of Monte Cristo, The Devil in the White City, The Great Bridge (Brooklyn Bridge), various biographies of famous people such as Einstein, Martin Luther, Steve Jobs, Elon Musk, and Benjamin Franklin.

I also spend time going to the Christian Businessman's Connection (CBMC) meetings. I meet with other Christian men weekly. I also go through the CBMC "Operation Timothy" program, which is a one-on-one discipleship program with other men.

I am a member of the Living Hope Church and participated as a collection counter once a month for several years. I also coordinated their Angel Tree program for several years.

Before Covid, I liked to go out to breakfast and lunch with friends.

I am also on the board of directors of M28 Ministry. M28 stands for Matthew 28. It is a one-on-one discipleship program that was established in 2011.

Houses

During my life, I lived in many houses. A brief summary follows.

195 Holmes St., Stratford, CT. From 1954 to 1973
I grew up in this house. We lived with my parents when we were newlyweds. Jen was born when we lived here.

64 Orchard St., Bridgeport, CT. From 1973 to 1974
When Jennifer was an infant, we rented a second-floor apartment in Bridgeport for about nine months. It was a 3-story house. We lived right around the corner from a Portuguese bakery. We would get fresh Portuguese rolls almost every day. Mrs. Gallo was our landlord. She lived on the first floor. At that time, I would carpool to college with Fred Vincent from 9 AM to noon. (Fred and I had all of our classes together for all four years of college.) Then I would come home for lunch, go to work at Nichols Engineering from 2 PM to 10 PM, do my college homework from 10:30 to midnight. The next day I would do the same routine.

66 Mohawk St., Stratford, CT. From 1974 to 1979
This was the first house that we purchased. We lived in this house when Karen and Danielle were born. We lived here when I graduated from college, studied for the CPA Exam , and passed it.

28 Falmouth St., Milford, CT. From Dec. 1979 to Feb. 1982

I joined the Milford Lions Club when we lived here. I have been a member of the Lions Club ever since. Terri joined the Milford Newcomers Club, where she met out lifelong friends Bob and Diane Rauch. We have wonderful memories with them. Terri was also an excellent racquetball player at the time. (I was not.)

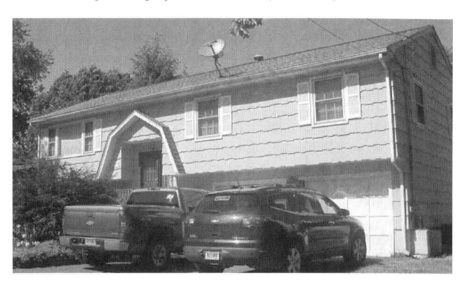

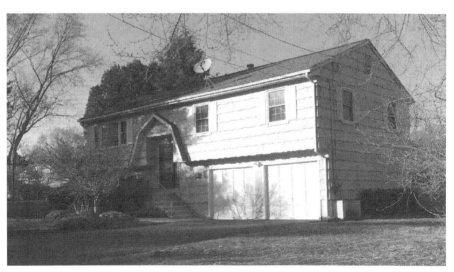

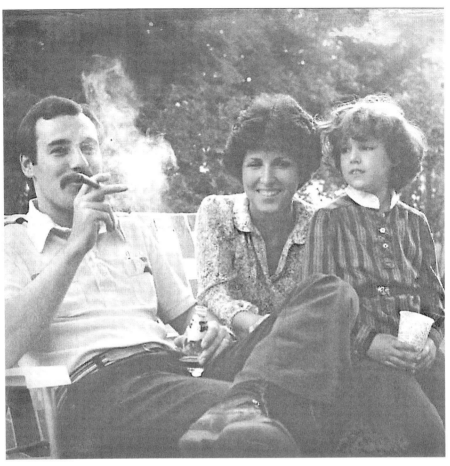

Dan, Terri, & Jennifer in the Rauch's backyard in Milford, CT

807 Hawley Ln., Stratford, CT. From Feb. 1982 to May 1987
Brittany was born while we lived in this house. She was seven weeks old when we moved to PA. Terri went to cosmetology school while we lived here and became a cosmetologist.

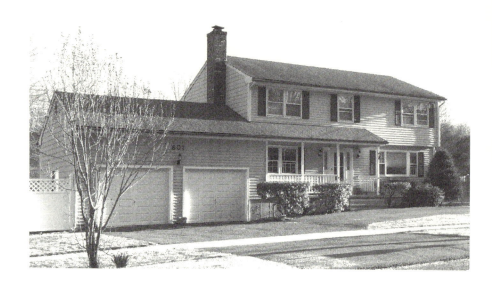

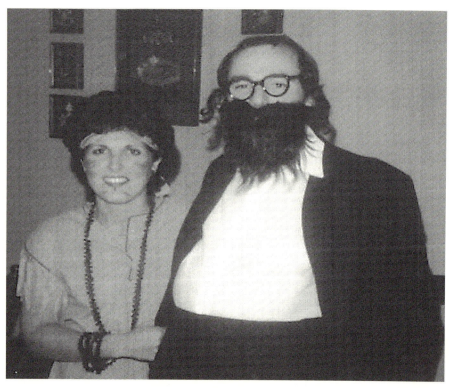

Terri and Dan in Halloween Costumes.

6115 Stephen's Crossing, Mechanicsburg, PA. From May 1987 to May 1997

This was our first house in Pennsylvania. Kelly was born when we lived in this house. Dr. Janson, our neighbor, delivered her.

20 Gunpowder Rd., Mechanicsburg, PA. From May 1997 to June 2002

We celebrated Y2K (the year 2000) with a black-tie family celebration at this house. We also had our 25th Wedding Anniversary in CT while we were living in this house. I surprised Terri with a gift of an almost new, silver Mazda Miata with a big red bow on it. For several years, I would cook a gourmet meal for the family. One that I remember is a lobster and pasta meal with Root Soup. (This was from a Martha Stewart cookbook.)

18501 Fontana Ln., Gaithersburg, MD. From June 2002 to October 2012

While we lived in MD, we were able to have the Miller Family live with us for several months. They were a family of 4, with two teenage boys. During that time, they were house hunting. I took the Metro to work in DC every day except for three days in 10 years. We lived about 3 miles from the Shady Grove Metro Station.

Summit Way, Mechanicsburg, PA. From October 2012 to Present

We moved here on October 19, 2012, shortly after I retired. Since we were involved while the house was being built, we had several amenities for handicapped people installed when we built the house, including an elevator. (see next page). We were also blessed to have the Romanacce family lived with us for several months. At that time, they were a family of 4. God has blessed them with two more children since then. During that time, they were house hunting.

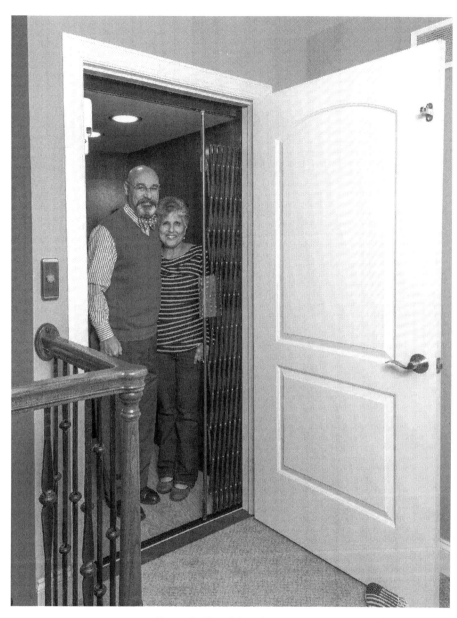

Dan & Terri in elevator

117 W. Vine St., Shiremanstown, PA. From 2005 to 2014
While we were living in Maryland, my parents had to go into nursing homes in Pennsylvania. Rather than pay for a hotel room to visit

them almost every weekend, we bought a small townhouse where we could stay on weekends while visiting them. When we moved back to PA, the Steinfield family lived in our townhouse from 2013 to 2014. Their family had two teenage boys. During that time, they were house hunting. The Peters family and my mother also lived in these townhouses while we were there.

Spanish Creek Drive, Ponte Vedra, FL. (Winter home) From November 2019 to Present

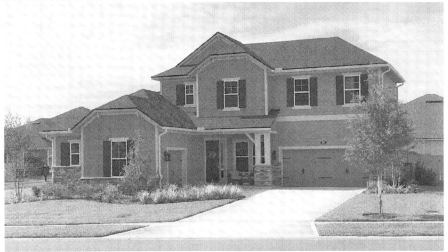

This house is directly across the street from the Boisvert family. We bought this house to avoid the winter ice and snow in PA so that we could be "snowbirds." The Boisvert's can watch the house while we are in PA, not being snowbirds. Because of Covid, the stay in FL has lasted a lot longer than three months.

KPMG - aka (Peat, Marwick, Mitchell & Co.)

White Plains, NY

I joined Peat, Marwick, Mitchell & Co. in White Plains, New York, in July 1976. My start date was 7/6/76. (That date was always easy to remember.) On that day, I met my lifelong friend, Nick Minissale.

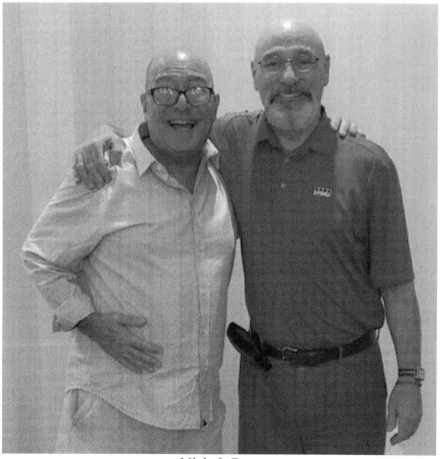

Nick & Dan

I began as an assistant accountant (auditor). I knew nothing about business except for what I had learned in college. That was probably a good thing because I started with a clean slate. I never did any tax returns. In my opinion, the rules are so onerous for tax returns and always changing that I never had the desire to do a tax return. I jokingly tell people that I would rather dig a ditch than do a tax return.

Throughout my career, I learned to be an excellent proofreader of financial reports and other documents. This proofreading skill came in handy when I would help my daughters while they were in school.

I ended up staying with the same firm for 37 years. I retired on September 30, 2013.

I joined Peat, Marwick, Mitchell & Co. in White Plains because it was the only CPA firm that offered me a job. (White Plains was 60 miles away from my house.). Several other firms rejected me.

Early in my career, after working many overtime hours and meeting clients' demanding, rigorous sign off dates on the audit of their financial statements, some audit teams would have a celebration dinner at a nice restaurant for every level of the audit team with spouses. A funny story about one of these dinners follows.

Terri and I could not attend one of these dinners. Several days after the dinner, I asked my team member if he and his wife had a good time at the dinner. He said, "yes," but he sat next to a very, very quiet team member. He told me that the quiet team member said three words to him all night. I asked him what those three words were. He replied that the other team member said, "pass the salt!" LOL

The name Peat, Marwick, Mitchell & Co. changed several times over the years that I was with the firm. It went from Peat, Marwick, Mitchell & Co. to KPMG Peat Marwick, to KPMG Peat and then to KPMG. KPMG stands for Klynvelt, Peat, Marwick, Goerdeler, the names of the founders of the firm. The firm began in 1897. When I joined the firm in 1976, it was known as one of the "Big 8" CPA firms. When I retired in 2012, only four of the Big 8 firms were left (the number was reduced through the merging of the big accounting firms.)

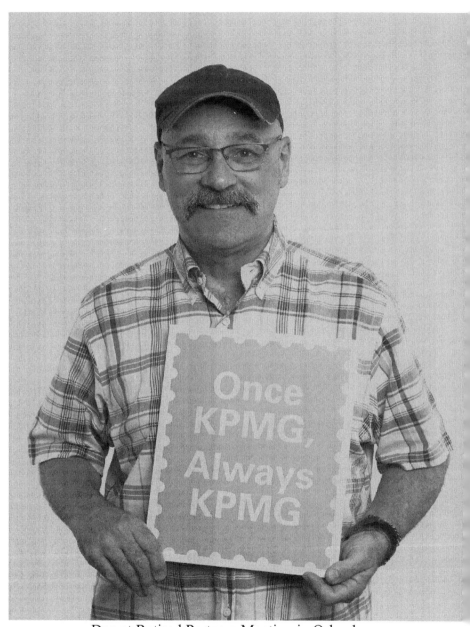
Dan at Retired Partners Meeting in Orlando

Stamford, CT

I was officially assigned to the Stamford, Connecticut office in 1980 when that office was opened. However, I spent most of my time with my clients and hardly ever went into the office.

My clients in the White Plains-Stamford office were Olin-Winchester, The General Signal Corp, GEO International, Tetley Inc., the Xerox Corporation, the Town of Fairfield, the Town of Greenwich, the Town of Weston, and various other clients.

Because of my government audit expertise, the vice-chairman of the government practice in our firm, Jack Miller, asked me if I would become the first Practice Fellow at the newly formed Governmental Accounting Standards Board (GASB).

This position was taken as a result of an agreement for me to come back to Peat Marwick in precisely two years. I interviewed for that position in 1984 and was employed by the GASB for two years from September 1, 1984 to August 31, 1986.

Harrisburg, PA

I transferred from the KPMG office in Stamford, CT to the KPMG office in Harrisburg, PA on May 1, 1987. The reason for my transfer was to perform the audit of the Commonwealth of Pennsylvania jointly with the Department of the Auditor General of the Commonwealth of Pennsylvania.

I was selected to work on that audit as a new partner. I was promoted from senior manager to partner on July 1, 1987. I transferred to the Harrisburg office at the suggestion of Jack Miller. Jack was one of my mentors.

KPMG audited the Commonwealth of Pennsylvania until 1995. Another firm underbid us at that time. Fortunately for me, I worked on the audits of several other government entities over the years, including school districts, counties, and cities. Because many of my clients were government clients, and the leaders were with different political parties, I never joined a political party. I tell people that I am not a Republican. I am not a Democrat. I am a Christian.

I then transferred to the manufacturing segment and gave all of my government clients to a new partner, Joe Seibert. The corporate clients that I audited included ShopVac Corporation, Precision Components Corporation, New World Pasta (a spin-off of Hershey Foods), Empire Kosher Poultry, Hanover Foods, Donsco (a foundry), Furman Foods, C-Cor Electronics Corporation, Nuclear Support Services, and Swatchwatch, (SMH).

On January 1, 1996, Dick Salus, the managing partner of the Harrisburg office, retired. On that date, I took over as the managing partner of the Harrisburg office. In that capacity, I reported to the managing partner of the Philadelphia office. Dick Salus was another one of my mentors.

In addition to my client responsibilities, my administrative duties included managing the Harrisburg office. Those administrative responsibilities included being actively involved in the community. Therefore, I was on the boards of the Pennsylvania Institute of Certified Public Accountants (PICPA), Bethesda Mission, Penn State-Harrisburg campus, the American Heart Association, and the United Way. I was also on the board of the Carlisle Country Club. During that time, I spent two years as President of the American Heart Association - Central Pennsylvania Chapter.

In 1997, KPMG celebrated its 100-year anniversary. We had various events throughout the year to celebrate. The firm had a 100-year anniversary logo made for the occasion.

I was at a PICPA conference in Lewisberry, PA, when the 911 crashes occurred on September 11, 2001. I went back to my office in Harrisburg at about 10 AM. Since our office was across the street from the Federal Courthouse, and we did not know the extent of the attacks, we sent everyone home for the day.

I started wearing a KPMG lapel pin around 1987. I wore it on my suit almost every day when we did not wear business casual clothing. We started wearing business casual clothing around 1992. One day I was on the elevator, and a stranger asked me whether KPMG was a radio station because most radio stations, west of the Mississippi River, start with the letter "K." LOL.

While I was in the Harrisburg and the WDC offices, I was one of only two partners in the country that were SEC Reviewing Partners for government "offering" documents.

Some of my favorite restaurants in the Harrisburg area include the Hershey Hotel, Alfred's Victorian, and the Union Canal House.

Washington DC

I started to work in the Washington DC office of KPMG in June 2002. Before that, I worked part-time in the Harrisburg office and part-time in the DC office for about six months.

Accounting for the federal government is different than accounting for local governments. Therefore, I had to learn accounting for the federal government by being the second partner on several engagements.

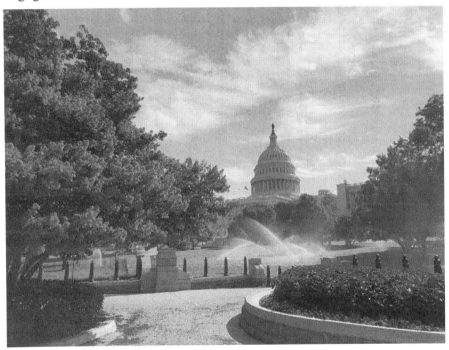

My clients included the Department of Commerce, the National Science Foundation, the newly-formed Transportation Security Administration, the Federal Bureau of Investigation (FBI), the Census

Bureau, the Patent and Trademark Office, and the National Institute of Standards and Technology.

After several years of federal accounting experience, I was assigned as the lead partner for the Department of the Treasury of the United States. This included the Community Development Financial Institutions Fund (CDFI) and the Treasury. The Treasury was my main client. Another client was the Commodities Futures Trading Commission. I was also the engagement partner, for three years, on the audit of the US Coast Guard, which is part of the Transportation Security Administration.

This was a good time to have the US Treasury for a client because this was when we had many financial issues in the United States. We worked very closely with the Treasury Inspector General's Office and the Government Accountability Office (GAO). We had many problems that had to be addressed that had never been addressed before, such as the bailout of some federal organizations.

My only local government client was the Washington Metropolitan Area Transit Authority (WMATA), the railroad system. I took the Metro Rail train into DC every day for ten years except for three days. I really enjoyed riding the Metro System.

While I worked in the DC office of KPMG, I also served on the Greater Washington Society of CPAs (GWSCPA) board of directors. During my term at the GWSCPAs, I worked closely on the "Mobility" issue.

I celebrated 25 years with the firm while I was in DC. I was recognized by the firm with a silver plate presented by the Managing Partner of the DC office. He later became Chairman of the entire firm, John Veihmeyer.

I received a Grandfathers' Clock for my 30th anniversary with the firm. I spent a total of 37 years with KPMG, including my two years as a practice fellow at GASB. I did not receive anything on my 35th Anniversary with the firm because the firm ended its recognition program by then. I retired on September 30, 2012. Even though I did not work with the firm from 2012 to 2013, I was considered disabled, which also counted as a year of service.

Near the end of my career, I was at an AICPA government conference in WDC on August 23, 2011. There was an earthquake in WDC. We had to evacuate the hotel in mid-afternoon.

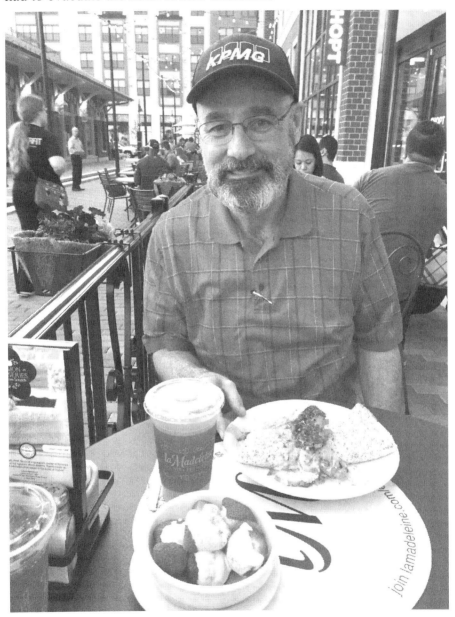

Marriage

Terri (Tereza) and I met at the Stratford Town Fair when I was 17, and she was 16. Terri is godly, kind, generous, loving, caring, compassionate, concerned with others' salvation, spontaneous, competitive, and beautiful. This was the first job for each of us. We dated for 13 months before we got married.

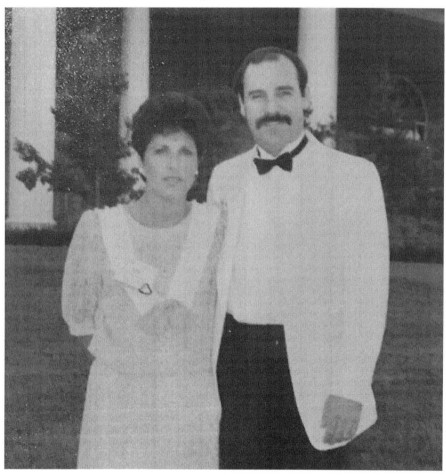

Terri & Dan

God has blessed us over the years with five daughters and 18 grandchildren. Many people say to me, "Wow, you have five girls, no boys?" My reply is usually "not yet." I follow up with Abraham's story in the Bible, who was approximately 100 when he had his son. There are not many people that have five girls and no boys. I calculate the percentage of that happening is 50% times 50% times 50% times 50% times 50%. That is around 3 in 100.

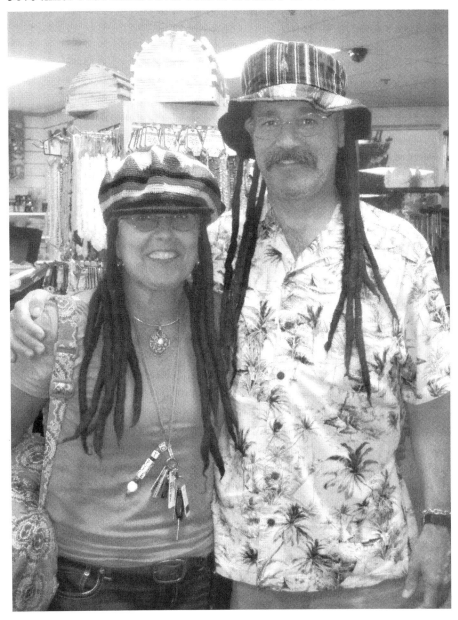

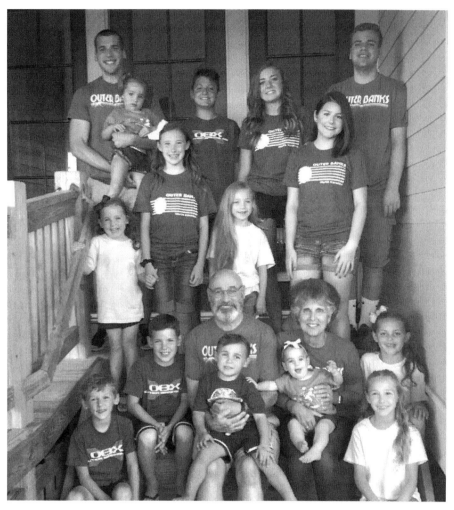

Dan, Terri, & most of the grandchildren

God has blessed us with many happy years of marriage.

I would not recommend a teenage marriage, but in our case, it was a blessing. After we got married, I worked full-time, and I went to college full-time. My schedule was as follows. I would go to college from 8 AM to 12 PM. Then, I would go home for lunch from 12 PM to 2 PM. I worked at a factory (Nichols Engineering Co.) from 2 PM to 10 PM. I would drive home from the factory from 10 PM to 10:30

PM. I would study for college from 10:30 PM until midnight. At midnight, I would go to sleep and begin the next day at approximately 7 AM in preparation for going to college at 8 AM.

Additionally, my wife, Terri, was a young mother. We were blessed by her having the support of her large family and because one of her sisters had a baby only three weeks earlier than ours. As new mothers, they did a lot of things together.

We also have five fantastic sons-in-law. I tell each of my sons-in-law that they are on my "top five" list of sons-in-law. At home, sometimes I would sing silly songs to Terri and the girls. The song I would sing to Terri was "Terri Baby" to the tune of "Sherry Baby" by Franky Valle and the Four Seasons, by changing Sherry to Terri throughout the song. Terri is also a gifted photographer. She has taken several college photography courses. She is also gifted by making creative Facebook posts.

For our 25th Wedding Anniversary, we renewed our wedding vows in Stratford Baptist Church. We had a best man and maid of honor, and we had a reception with about 100 people at the Hilton Hotel in Stratford, CT, in 1998.

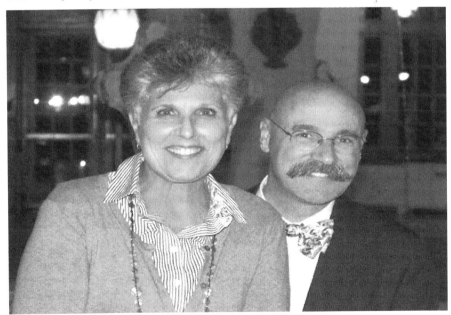

For our 46th Anniversary, Terri surprised me with celebratory lawn signs and ornaments.

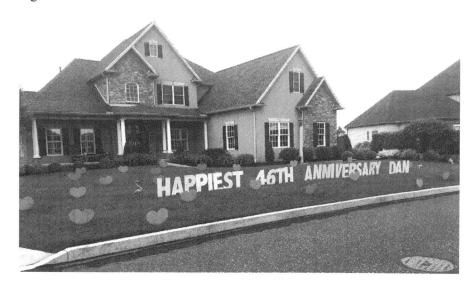

Memory Verses

I firmly believe that memorizing key verses in the Bible helps us grow closer to God.

Over the years, I have memorized several Bible verses and passages. This list is not all-inclusive. Many of these verses I memorized in my retirement.

Psalm 1, Psalm 63, Psalm 19 - My Golden Psalm (The psalm that matches the day of my birthday.) and Psalm 150.

Psalm 19:14, (my words and meditations)

Psalm 24:7, (the King of Glory),

Psalm 119:67, and Psalm 119:71, (afflictions),

Matthew 5:3-11, (the Beatitudes),

2 Corinthians 5:20-21, (Christ's Ambassador),

2 Corinthians 4:16-18, (afflictions),

Galatians 5:22-23 (fruits of the Spirit),

Ephesians 4:29 (uplifting speech)

Ephesians 6:10-20, (the armor of God),

James, Chapter 1,

3 John 4, (children)

Some of these verses relate to "afflictions." As we all get older, these verses become more important to us.

Morning Routine

This chapter will be helpful to those that have SCA.

In the morning, I generally wake up around 6:30 AM. I usually listen to an hour-long sermon by John MacArthur by using the Grace To You app on the phone. He has been preaching for over 50 years. The sermons are by topic as well as by books of the Bible. The Grace to You app has a tremendous number of resources available for free.

In addition to listening to a sermon each morning, I make a cup of coffee using my Keurig coffee maker, which is in the master bathroom. I wear rubber shoes, which help me not to slip or fall down in the morning when I'm getting ready.

We also have handicap bars in the bathroom and the shower area. These bars can be permanently installed, or you can buy temporary ones from Bed, Bath, and Beyond, etc. I also shave with an electric razor. It is less likely that I will be cut with an electric razor than with a straight-edge razor.

I also have two plastic handicap chairs. One is in the shower area because the shower area is rather big. The second one is outside of the shower area in the place where I prepare for the day. The chairs also act as handicapped bars. They can be moved. They also help with my balance.

I do not have any throw rugs in the house. This is a good suggestion for everyone, even those that don't have a balance problem. I use Velcro shoes and a Velcro watchband. It is easier than tying shoes or using a regular watch band.

I take the following vitamin supplements: Vitamin D 3, biotin, and magnesium 4000 MCG (to avoid muscle cramps throughout my body). The only prescription drug that I have right now is Omeprazole 20. That is to prevent heartburn. I take one of those in the morning and one in the evening. I also take the magnesium in the morning and the evening.

If I am not ready for the day when the sermon ends, I listen to Christian music. My favorites songs are from Sovereign Grace Music,

Elvis gospel, Don Marsh gospel music, Johnny Cash gospel music, Alan Jackson gospel music, and the Inspirations.

I also use Alexa in the morning for an alarm, to get the weather in any city in the United States, for a timer, to communicate with others with an Alexa, to add items to my shopping list or create other lists, to tell me what is on my calendar for the day, to turn off and turn on the lights, to get the joke of the day, to get the day in history, to read Kindle books, and to read Audible books.

I also ask Alexa various questions throughout the day.

Nichols Engineering

In June 1973, a friend of mine suggested that I join the work crew on the third shift (11 PM to 7 AM) at Nichols Engineering. The company made rubber goods made to engineering specifications.

My first job there was as a mold operator. I describe this as operating four huge waffle irons, one at a time (approximately 24" x 24"). When one was done (cured), the next one was ready to be opened. The large waffle irons were called molds. These molds would have four cavities, with precise markings, in each mold. They were for large "O" rings around 8 inches in diameter. The rubber was put into the cavities; the mold was shut and then pushed into the ovens. They would be in the ovens for approximately 15 minutes and then taken out. The process would start all over with the next mold.

This lasted for an eight-hour shift. The mold room was sweltering. It was close to 100°. Because it was the middle of the summer, it was very hot. Obviously, the mold room was not air-conditioned. We had to wear insulated gloves to handle the molds. We often burnt ourselves on our wrists or lower arms.

My brother, brothers-in-law, and numerous friends also got jobs there that summer.

In August, the plant was shut down for a week in order to maintain it. This meant cleaning the rubber gunk out of all of the machines and throughout the factory. While I was working during "shut down," the machine shop boss asked me if I would help him. I said, "yes."

The machine shop was immaculate as compared to the mold room. It had an average temperature. Therefore, I thought if I did a good job, they might want to keep me in the machine shop. Thanks be to God, he let me stay in the machine shop.

My new boss was fantastic. He let me adjust my working hours to be from 2 PM to 10 PM so I could go home and study. The rest of the factory worked from 3 PM to 11 PM. When times were tough and people were getting laid off, he allowed me to work on Saturdays to earn a little extra money.

If it wasn't for him, I don't think I would have been able to complete college.

God blessed me by being offered to stay in the machine shop to work. I worked there for the rest of my time at college. (Approximately three years.)

Several years ago, I went back to the site of the factory. The factory is no longer there. A hotel is there now.

Non-profit Organizations

In 1979, I joined the Bridgeport Chapter of the National Association of Accountants (NAA) and the Milford Lions Club.

I was the president of the Bridgeport Chapter of the National Association of Accountants around 1983. Before that, I served in various board positions. I was a member of these two organizations until I moved to the Harrisburg, Pennsylvania area in 1987.

In 1984 and 1985, I was the President of the Milford Lions Club (2 terms). After being President, I became a Zone Chairman for one year, then Deputy District Governor for one year. I worked closely with Roland Ladd. I kept my membership in the Lions Club wherever I moved. I have been a Lion for over 40 years.

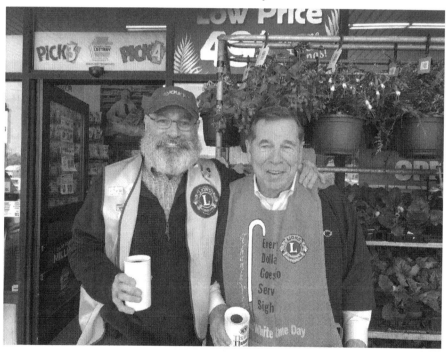

Lions Club White Cane Day Collections

When I retired, I saw Jim Wolfe at breakfast one day. He invited me to attend a Harrisburg Lions Club meeting. I have attended and been active ever since. I became the Treasurer around 2014. This includes doing accounting and paying bills.

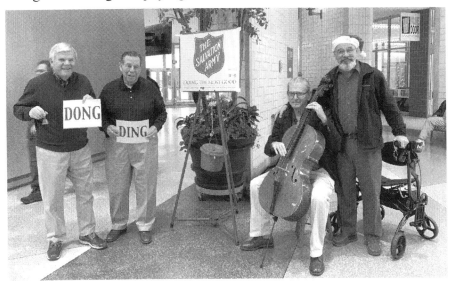

Lions Club Salvation Army Collections

I am still the Treasurer. I issue financial statements for the Harrisburg Lions Club every month. I also made the financial statements easier to understand. I developed two spreadsheets that I use for the Lions Club. One is linked to the other, so when I input the monthly activity, it will automatically show the year-to-date activity. The revised totals will be shown in the monthly financial statements automatically.

Since we have not had Lions Club meetings due to the coronavirus, we have been having virtual meetings using Zoom. In addition to my Treasurer functions, I participate in most Lions' fund-raising events, including pancake breakfasts and White Cane Days.

I transferred to the Harrisburg Lions Club in 1988. As mentioned earlier, I joined various other organizations while I was a partner in Harrisburg. (See KPMG - Harrisburg section of this book.) I was also active with Christian Business Men's Connection (CBMC).

Although I was not a board member for the Whitaker Center, I helped to raise funds to build its new facility across the street from my office. I organized "The CPA Challenge."

I was a member of the American Institute of CPAs (AICPA) since 1979. Over the years, I taught a 2-day course for the AICPA on "Government Auditing Standards." I had my choice where and when I would teach it. Some of the locations were San Juan, Los Angeles, the Robert Morris College near Pittsburgh, and Voorhees, NJ.

When I moved to the Washington DC area, I remained a member of the Harrisburg Lions Club. However, I was unable to attend any meetings. While in the DC area, I joined the Association of Government Accountants and was extremely active with the Greater Washington Society of CPAs. I helped with the "Mobility" legislation.

For several years, in the latter part of my career, I also wrote CPA Exam questions about government accounting and auditing.

Although my physical activity is limited, we like to support a number of non-profit organizations. Most of our contributions are to Christian organizations.

They include Christian Business Men's Connection (CBMC), M28 Ministry, China Outreach Ministries, Bethesda Mission, The PA Family Institute, Disciple Makers, Campus Ambassadors, The Bible League, Christian Schools of Greater Harrisburg, Finish The Mission 2030 (mission to Nepal), Museum of the Bible, several churches, and the Lions Club of Harrisburg.

I am on the Boards of Directors of M28 Ministry and the Lions Club of Harrisburg. I also learned how to use merge mail for some Lions Club needs and for the Angel Tree project that I worked on. I like to try to make things as efficient as possible.

Since we strongly believe in Christian education, we continue to invest in the Christian Schools of Greater Harrisburg and have set up a scholarship fund there.

Number Facts

Because I like numbers, number games, number puzzles, etc. and since I was a CPA for many years, I have included this chapter.

Our 13th grandchild was born on 6/7/13. 6 + 7 =13. Her brother was born on 6/9/15. 6 + 9 = 15. (But he was the 14th grandchild.)

My mother's only grandson was born on February 4. Her 1st great-grandson was born 16 years later on February 4. Our youngest daughter and our oldest granddaughter were both born on September 29.

I started my career at KPMG on July 6, 1976. (7-6-7-6)

One of my grandfathers died exactly one week after my brother's birthday, and the other grandfather died exactly one week after my birthday.

My father lived for 76 years and three days. His sister, my aunt, lived 76 years and two days. (She was 18 years older than him.)

There are 66 chapters in the book of Isaiah in the Bible. The first 39 chapters focus on the time before Jesus. The last 27 chapters focus on Jesus. The book of Isaiah was written about 700 years before the birth of Jesus.

There are 66 books in the Bible. The first 39 are in the Old Testament, which was written to describe the time before Jesus was born, and the last 27 books are in the New Testament, which focuses on Jesus's life.

God named one of the books in the Bible "Numbers."

Pets

When I was a little boy, we had a small black dog with long hair. She was part cocker spaniel. Her name was Suzy. My mother always liked the name Suzy but never had any girls to use it. So, she used it for our dog. We also had several hamsters. My brother also had some small turtles.

When I was about 13, Susie died. We got a new puppy named Amos. We had him for several months, then he got hit by a car and died. We then got another female dog. She had one litter of puppies. We kept one of the puppies. The mother dog's name was Becky, and the puppy was named Winnie. My parents had those dogs for over ten years.

In our 20s, when our kids were little, we had a very big dog. He was a mix between a Belgian Shepherd and a Golden Retriever. We had him for about 14 years.

We then got a Sheltie from my parent's litter of puppies. The Sheltie was named Lady Liberty. We had Lady for about ten years and then gave her away.

We did not have any animals for about ten years. In 2010, we got a Cockapoo named Tootie. Tootie came to us from St. Louis. The youngest daughter in the movie "Meet Me in St. Louis" was named Tootie. Thus, we called the dog Tootie. Tootie lived for seven years. She had a painful back issue and had to be put to sleep.

We got Tati (short for Tatiana), another Cockapoo, in 2017. (Tatiana was one of the daughters that was discussed in the book about the Romanov Family in Russia.)

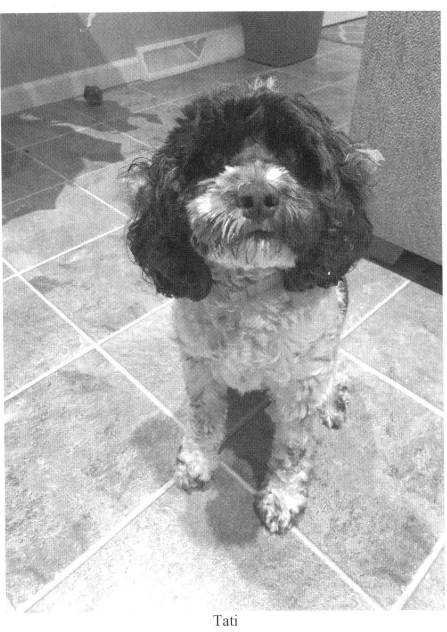
Tati

Publications

Over the years, I wrote several accounting items that were published. They include:

Understanding your Town's Financial Statements. (approximately 1985)

SOX-Will it fit? (A KPMG publication around 2003)

Governmental Accounting Standards Board Statement (GASB) 3, Reporting on Repurchase Agreements. (1985)

Measurement Focus/Basis of Accounting Exposure Draft – GASB publication (1986)

Quotes

John Newton

The most significant problem we face as a nation is our sin, and the only ultimate solution is Christ crucified!

I am not what I ought to be, I am not what I want to be, I am not what I hope to be in another world; but still, I am not what I once used to be, and by the grace of God, I am what I am.

Unknown

Have you ever noticed that anyone going slower than you is an idiot, but anyone going faster is a maniac?

We take photos as a return ticket to a moment otherwise gone!

We can open our mouths, but only God can open the heart.

Where the Scriptures speak, discussion ceases; where the scriptures do not speak, discussion is useless.

Grace Gems

You may go to Heaven . . . without health, without wealth, without honor, without pleasure, without friends, without learning, but you can never go to Heaven without Christ! "I am the way and the truth and the life. No one comes to the Father except through Me." John 14:6

Spurgeon

The Bible will lead you from sin, OR sin will lead you from the Bible.

John Owen

He that hath slight thoughts of sin never had great thoughts of God.

Ruth Bell Graham

One day, Billy Graham and Ruth were driving on a highway. They saw a sign that said "End of Construction --- Thank you for your patience." She liked that saying so much, she had it put on her gravestone.

God's Not Dead 2

I'd rather stand with God and be judged by the world than stand with the world and be judged by God.

Martin Luther

I have so much to do that I shall spend the first three hours in prayer.

Charles Spurgeon, Checkbook of Faith, 6/04

If Jesus were to listen to your talk, would he be pleased with it?

Thomas Manton, Works, 1:1 67-173

When you fly from God as a friend, you fly to him as judge!

John Knox speaking of the days during the Reformation.

God gave his Holy Spirit to simple man in great abundance.

John Bunyan

You can do more than pray after you have prayed, but you cannot do more than pray until you have prayed.

Thomas Watson, Voices From The Past, Vol. 2, p. 67

Mercy is an innate propensity in God to do good to distressed sinners.

Richard Baxter, Voices From The Past, Vol. 1, p. 311

Christ came from Heaven that we might go to Heaven.

Restaurants, Amusement Parks, & Museums

Restaurants

Some of my favorite restaurants are: The Palm, Morton's Steakhouse, Ruth Chris Steak House, Alfred's Victorian, the Hershey Hotel, The Columbia (various locations in Florida)

My favorite meal is Filet Mignon with Bearnaise Sauce (cooked medium well), Mashed Potatoes with Gravy, Onion Rings, and Tiramisu. I also like almost every type of Italian food. I do not like any seafood.

Amusement Parks

Rye Playland, as a child

Hershey Park - numerous times

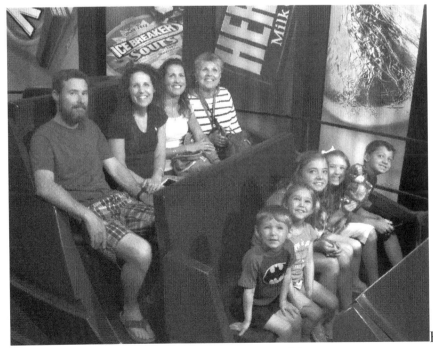

Hershey Chocolate World

Museums

The Holocaust Museum, the Museum of the Bible, the National Geographic Museum, The Newseum, The Corcoran Gallery of Art, The Smithsonian Museums, including the Air & Space Museum, Thomas the Train Museum in Strasburg, PA

Other Places of Interest

Arlington Cemetery, the Kennedy Center, the Watergate Hotel, the Washington Nationals Baseball Park, The Washington Convention Center, Chinatown, the Treasury building, the White House, The Washington Monument, the Lincoln Memorial, the Cherry Blossom Festival, Fords Theater, Constitution Hall, The Metro System, Ollie's Trolley Restaurant,

Sight and Sound Live Theater - Strasburg, PA, The Whitaker Center - Harrisburg, PA

Salvation

This is the most important chapter of this book.

I got saved around 1973. My brother came home for a summer break from Moody Bible Institute and witnessed to each one of us in our family. He used the Roman Road and Revelation 3:20.

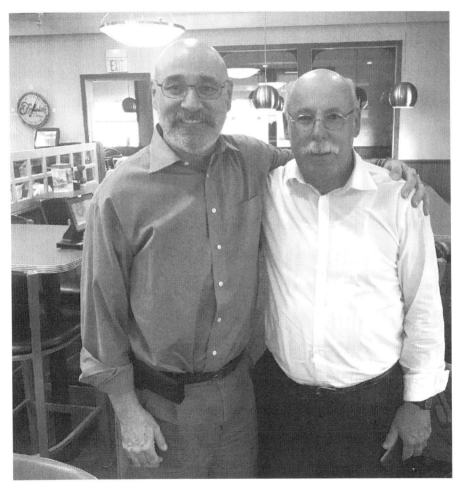

Brothers 2019

Shortly after that, we joined Stratford Baptist Church. My parents and Terri were also saved around the same time. We all were baptized together around 1973. Subsequently, we had a group of young adults studying the Bible at our home.

By salvation, I mean that we were saved from eternal Hell and obtained the free gift of eternal life in Heaven. This is clearly written in the Bible.

Believing in Jesus is the ONLY way to go to heaven.

In the Bible, verse John 14:6 says.

Jesus said to him, "I am **the** way, and the truth, and the life. No one comes to the Father except through me.

John 3:16 says:

For God so loved the world, that he gave his only Son, that whoever believes in him should not perish but have eternal life.

By the word "witnessed," I mean that my brother talked to each of us individually and explained the only way to salvation is to believe that Jesus Christ paid the penalty of our sins by dying for those who believe, according to the Bible.

When I said the "Roman Road," my brother used five verses from the book of Romans, which is in the Bible, to convey this message of salvation to us.

Those verses are Romans 3:10, Romans 3:23, Romans 5:8, Romans 6:23, and Romans 10:9.

Romans 3:10. "as it is written: None is righteous, no, not one;"

Romans 3:23. "for all have sinned and fall short of the glory of God."

Romans 5:8. "but God shows his love for us in that while we were still sinners, Christ died for us."

Romans 6:23. "For the wages of sin is death, but the free gift of God is eternal life in Christ Jesus our Lord."

Romans 10:9. "because, if you confess with your mouth that Jesus is Lord and believe in your heart that God raised him from the dead, you will be saved."

My brother also demonstrated this by the verse from Revelation 3:20, which is Jesus knocking at a door, and if you are willing to open the door to let Jesus into your life, he will give you salvation.

Revelation 3:20 says. "Behold, I stand at the door and knock. If anyone hears my voice and opens the door, I will come in to him and eat with him, and he with me."

The Bible clearly says that we do not get saved by our good works. I thought this before I started to read the Bible and listen to sermons from Bible-believing churches. Many people believe that they will go to Heaven by doing good works. According to the Bible, this is not true.

However, once someone is saved, that person wants to do good deeds. By doing good deeds, this is acting like Jesus acted when he was on earth.

If you have not been "saved," you must be saved to have life forever in heaven.

When you accept Jesus as your Savior, that is called justification. It is a one-time event.

Sanctification is a lifelong process (a lifelong challenge) to be righteous and Christ-like in everything that you do for the rest of your life. We work on sanctification for the rest of our lives, but we will never be completely sinless, no matter how hard we try. Only Christ was, and is, completely sinless.

According to the Bible, if you don't go to Heaven forever, you go to Hell forever. There is no in-between. You either accept Jesus as your Savior and go to Heaven for eternity, or you do not accept Jesus as your Savior and go to Hell forever.

I pray that you choose the former.

One of my favorite Bible verses is from 3 John 4, "I have no greater joy than to hear that my children are walking in the truth."

There are numerous ways to grow spiritually, such as going to Christian conferences, which include Together for the Gospel (T4G), the Banner of Truth, and the Christian Business Men's Connection.

You will also need to regularly attend a Bible-believing church, pray, study, and read the Bible.

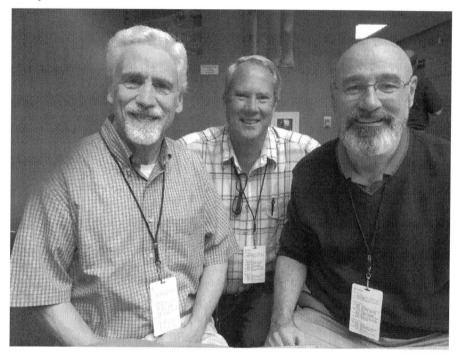

Banner of Truth Conference

John Adams, the second President of the United States said: "Suppose a nation in some distant region should take the Bible for their only law book, and every member should regulate his conduct by the precepts there exhibited! ... what a paradise would this region be."

Why do I believe the Bible is true?

The Bible was written (inspired) by the Holy Spirit (God), physically written by 40 different writers over 1,500 years on three continents in three different languages. A consistent, complete message unfolds across its pages. The Bible is a composition of 66 books (39 books in the Old Testament and 27 books in the New Testament.) The Old Testament describes what happened in the world before Jesus Christ was born. The New Testament focuses on the birth of Jesus, his life, and the future.

The reason why I believe the Bible is true is summarized nicely in a quote that is on page 19 of Book 1 of CBMC's Operation Timothy – Questions. This is a quote from Hugh Ross, astrophysicist, www.reason.org.

"Approximately 2,500 prophecies appear in the Bible, about 2,000 of which already have been fulfilled to the letter – no errors. Since the probability for any one of these prophecies having been fulfilled by chance averages less than one in ten, and since the prophecies are for the most part independent of one another, the odds for all these prophecies having been fulfilled by chance without error is less than one in 10 to the 2,000 power!"

For example, the book of Isaiah (Isaiah 7:14), in the Bible, prophesied that Jesus would be born of a virgin 700 years before he was born. There was never a virgin birth before or since the birth of Jesus.

"Eternal" and "eternity" are difficult words to truly understand. The lyrics in the song "Amazing Grace," give me the right perspective. It says: about heaven:

"…When we've been there ten thousand years,

Bright shining as the sun,

We've no less days to sing God's praise

Than, when we'd first begun."

I have heard unsaved people described as "pre-Christians." I believe this term is very accurate because anyone can become a Christian up to their point of death.

C. S. Lewis, a great author, and Atheist turned Christian, said that based on the Bible, "Jesus is either a liar, a lunatic, or Lord." He is absolutely correct.

Another one of his quotes follows.

Christianity, if false, is of no importance, and if true, of infinite importance. The only thing It cannot be is moderately important.

To me, one of the most important characters in the New Testament in the Bible is the thief on the cross next to Jesus.

Their conversation follows:

39 One of the criminals who were hanged railed at him, saying, "Are you not the Christ? Save yourself and us!"

40 But the other rebuked him, saying, "Do you not fear God, since you are under the same sentence of condemnation?

41 And we indeed justly, for we are receiving the due reward of our deeds; but this man has done nothing wrong."

42 And he said, "Jesus, remember me when you come into your kingdom."

43 And he said to him, "Truly, I say to you, today you will be with me in paradise." (Luke 23:39-43)

This clearly proves that you do not get to Heaven by doing good deeds. The thief did not have a chance to do any good deeds but Jesus promised to see him in paradise that day!

Your new life should begin with a simple prayer similar to the one that follows.

Dear Lord Jesus, I know that I am a sinner, and I ask for Your forgiveness. I believe You died for my sins and rose from the dead. I turn from my sins and invite You to come into my heart and life. I want to trust and follow You as my Lord and Savior. In Your Name. Amen.

Sovereign Grace

We believe that God blessed us to be at Covenant Life Church at the right time in the church's life. CJ Mahaney was the lead pastor, and there were approximately 15 other pastors. CJ is one of the best preachers I have ever heard. The youth group was at its best. Brittany and Kelly both participated.

They also graduated from Covenant Life Christian School. In their senior years, I went with each of them to Juarez, Mexico, to do missionary work. Those trips were fantastic opportunities.

I also participated in the "Invest" course, which was led by Pastor Robin Boisvert. Brittany married Robin's third son after they graduated from the University of Maryland. Terri and I also participated in several sessions of the "Alpha" group.

After several years, CJ resigned as lead pastor, and Josh Harris took over as lead pastor. The church had over 1,000 members. (Josh was the author of several Christian books, including "I Kissed Dating Goodbye.")

We joined the church just after the new portion of the church building was opened. During the ten years that we were at the church, we participated in several "Care Groups." Raul Pons led the first one. We made several life-long friends at the church. As a result of being associated with the church, the Christian school, and the Care Groups, we grew as Christians more in the ten years we were there than we did in the prior 30 years.

In the last two years that we lived in Maryland, 2010-2012, I also participated in the CBMC group that met in Gaithersburg, Maryland.

Spinocerebellar Ataxia (SCA)

I was diagnosed with SCA in May 2010. I was taking an annual physical, and the doctor had me touch my nose and then touch his finger. Because I was not entirely accurate, he sent me to a neurologist for an MRI. I had the MRI, and a week or so later, the neurologist called me in to tell me that I have SCA.

I was not surprised since my father had it, two of his brothers had it, and we believe his mother had it. One of his cousins also had SCA. I also have two cousins and one second cousin that have it right now. Those cousins are located in San Francisco, Scotland, and Connecticut. They are all in their late 50s to early 60s. The type of SCA that I have starts showing symptoms around age 55.

There is an excellent article about SCA on Wikipedia. (See Appendix 1.) They have done much research since my father had it. They say there are around 40 different types of SCA now.

When my father had it from 1987 through 2006, they called the disease Olivopontocerebellum Atrophy (rarediseases.org.)

When I lived in Maryland, someone that went to our church worked at the National Institute of Health (NIH). As a result, I set up an appointment with NIH. They were interested in the genetics of the disease and the relatives that also have it. Since there is no treatment, nor is there a cure, I have not been to NIH in a while.

The types that I have are type 1 and type 8. I had to get a blood test to determine what type I had. There are very few people that have SCA. Since I have two different types, NIH experts believe that I received one type from my mother and one type from my father. This is very, very unusual. NIH tested my mother before her death. She had an abundance of SCA 8, but exhibited no characteristics.

My father exhibited all the characteristics and ultimately died as a result of SCA.

To get hereditary SCA, you have to get the gene from one of your parents. I have one brother, and he does not have SCA. My cousins that have it have two other siblings that do not have it. Therefore, 50% of the siblings got SCA. In my second cousin's immediate family, two of the eight siblings got SCA. However, some have not yet reached age 55.

There is an Ataxia unit at the Johns Hopkins University. I participated in a cognitive study with them for two years. However, the funding ran out, and I no longer go there. They have an Ataxia Focus Group that offers excellent webinars for free.

There is an excellent movie on someone with a different type of Ataxia called "The Ataxian." This shows a person in their 20s who was a team member who rode their bicycles across the country. It is very interesting, and it shows that people with Ataxia can participate in certain events.

When I was first diagnosed with Ataxia, my neurologist said, "Do as much as you can as long as you can." This is good advice.

As I said, there are many different types of Ataxia. Some types affect children, some types affect young adults, and some types affect older adults. The type that I have affects older adults. Since the type that I have affects older adults, most of my life was lived without SCA. Fortunately, SCA is not painful. It only becomes painful when you fall and break something.

I use a Rollator now, which is a walker with wheels. I have been using that for about two years. Before that, I used a cane for about three years to help with my balance. To make my affliction fun for the grandchildren, I asked each family to pick a unique walking cane out of the Fashionable Canes brochure. I also give the smaller grandchildren fun rides on the seat of the rollator. Eventually, I will "graduate" to a wheelchair. Then finally to bed rest.

Most people, when they see that you are handicapped, treat you very nicely. They hold doors for you and accommodate you when they are nearby.

One thing that I have found out is that you must go slow in whatever you are doing. You must minimize physical activity, except for safe exercise. The exercise that I did was to exercise in a unique physical therapy water pool under physical therapists' guidance. If you fall in a water pool, you will not be hurt. I also had a physical therapist helping with exercises that don't require balance at the YMCA.

Because we are sheltering in place due to the coronavirus, I bought a stationary recumbent bicycle that I can use in the home to continue my exercise. The exercise isn't as rigorous as the YMCA, but it is better than nothing. The YMCA closed temporarily for the coronavirus issues.

When I was diagnosed with the disease, I said I should have chronicled my father's disease progression when he was living. The neurologist at NIH told me that this disease affects everyone slightly differently, and therefore that would not have been a big help. Since I did not see my father daily, and he did not speak much about himself, I did not know much about SCA until I started getting the symptoms. I hope this book will be helpful with other family members that get SCA.

Another good thing about this affliction is that it does not affect cognitive abilities. Although I have become more emotional as I got older, I don't know if this relates to my SCA. I got very emotional giving speeches at my father's wake, at my mother's funeral, at my retirement party in the KPMG WDC office, and my retirement party at the Trump National Golf Club in Virginia. My grandson, Brian Peters Jr., read my mother's eulogy for me, and he read my retirement speech for me at the Trump National Golf Club.

I also did one month of experimental hyperbaric oxygen treatments. Since this was experimental, it was not covered by insurance. I did not notice any improvements during the month that I had these treatments. If I had done it longer, maybe I would have seen some progress. The treatments were expensive.

Other than SCA, I am very healthy, thank God. I tell people that I feel like I am 25 years old. My cholesterol is around 200; my heartbeat is about 75, I have no aches or pains, no cancer, no heart issues, no high blood pressure, no hearing issues, and no arthritis. I am very blessed. Over the years, I have had no stitches, no hernias, and no significant operations. I had the following procedures: Tonsils and adenoids removed (age 3), arthroscopic gall bladder removed (age 46).

Even if you have a disease that affects a part of your body, you should not neglect the rest of your body. Get an annual physical examination, get a yearly blood test, get a flu shot, get a colonoscopy, exercise, control your weight, etc.

I take several supplements: vitamin D3, magnesium (to prevent muscle cramps), and biotin. The only prescription drug that I take is Omeprazole 20 twice each day to prevent heartburn.

Some Things I Have Learned Relating to SCA

The Apple Watch 4 and newer can detect a fall and automatically calls emergency telephone numbers for you.

Slow down. Doing things fast may result in a fall with long-term damage.

Do as much as you can as long as you can. (advice from the neurologist)

Don't try to multitask. (Do one thing at a time.)

Get a "Permanently Disabled" car license plate and a portable placard for a second or third car. I also try to park my car near the shopping cart stalls. I can then use the shopping cart as a walker.

Get a health bracelet with your name on it, the name of the disease, and a description of the conditions (slurring, loss of balance). If you don't have one and a police officer stops you, he/she might think you are drunk.

Because I have difficulty writing and printing, I use electronic checks for the Lions Club and personally. Most of my payments are made electronically, but I use Deluxe Checks Corporation when I want to write a check electronically.

Use the KISS method as much as possible. The KISS Method is the Keep It Simple System.

Accept help from others when they offer to help. (People like to help others.)

ALWAYS say "thank you" even for the smallest things.

Use the rollator seat to transport items throughout the house. Put your food tray on the rollator seat in a buffet line.

Put a cup holder on your rollator. Always cover your drinks tightly, so they don't spill as you use the rollator.

I memorized my credit card number to order things online without having to get up and get my credit card out of my wallet every time I ordered something using my credit card. This has been useful numerous times.

Because I have difficulty writing cursive and block letters, I usually type my addresses and return addresses, print them, cut them out, and tape them to my envelopes. I keep a file for addresses on my computer, so they are available when I want to use that address in the future. (My computer typing has about 75% error, so I have to proofread carefully and make many revisilna. (revisions). (That was an example! LOL)

One of the most important things is to have grab bars in the bathroom/shower area. They can be permanently installed, or they can be portable ones that use strong suction on tile or glass. I also have two pairs of rubber shoes to prevent slipping on the bathroom and shower floor. I have two sets, which allows one to completely dry while I wear the other pair the next day.

Therapies

I went to 3 different types of therapy: physical therapy, speech therapy, and occupational therapy.

Physical therapy

For several months, I worked with an aquatic physical therapist. She developed various exercises I can do in the pool. These exercises concentrate on using my core. By using the core more, it will improve my balance.

The aquatic therapy pool is very different from a regular swimming pool. A normal swimming pool is about 3 feet deep and then slopes to about 8 feet deep. The aquatic therapy pool has four lanes. Each lane has a different depth starting with 4 feet, 4'6", 5 feet, and 5'6". Now that I know all the exercises, I do them in the pool by myself, without a physical therapist present. I believe it helps my balance to some extent. However, the real benefit is getting exercise for 1.5 hours for three days a week. When I walk on dry land, I find it helpful to concentrate on my core and keep my eyes fixed on an object far away. The focus is on the distant object rather than right in front of me. If I look down in front of me, there is a good chance I will fall.

Speech therapy

I do have some slurring when I speak. I also talk very slowly. I had six sessions with speech therapists. They helped with several improvements regarding my speech. Among them were slowing down, enunciating words properly, speaking closer to the individual, not talking with noise in the background, practicing tongue twisters, and reading out loud. Reading sentences out loud that focus on particular types of words, for example, S words or SH words, long words, or short phrases, which I tend to blend together, will help me with my speech.

Occupational therapy

I had about five visits with occupational therapists. They helped me with my daily activities. They introduced me to several different "gadgets" that will help me as I lose my motor skills. They introduced me to exercises that I can do with my cane. They also introduced me to activities that I can do with large rubber bands and to keep my muscles in shape.

They showed me weights for my pen, which will help me write a little neater. They suggested I continue to use dictation for my typing needs. The Occupational Therapists also gave me a therapeutic putty to use to make my hands stronger. They agreed that using a backpack is smart. I can concentrate on using my hands to stabilize my walking rather than carrying things. Also, using a tray placed on my rollator's seat can help move multiple food items at a single time.

They also gave me a brochure with a tremendous number of items that can be used for handicapped people. As the need arises, I will purchase some of these items. They also introduced me to a rubber, sticky pad that is used to untwist tops to bottles and jars. They are called DYCEN pads.

I use a button threader. This is a handheld gadget with a wire attached. You put the wire through buttonholes, then attach it to small buttons and pull the button back through the buttonhole. This gadget is useful when you know how to use it.

I purchased a ruler/magnifying glass to help me read. This ruler highlights the line that I'm reading, and it also magnifies the line. I also use the magnifying glass app on my phone for print that is too small to read on bottles, instructions, etc.

I use the Amazon Alexa along with the Smart Home plugs to turn lights on for me verbally. This is good for getting up at night and not hunting for the light switch and falling as a result. A stylus is also helpful in improving accuracy for typing on the cell phone. Additionally, speech recognition software is good instead of typing on the computer.

I can go back to each of these therapists and have a benchmark test to gauge how much I have lost motor skills.

Travel

As I mentioned earlier, I traveled an appropriate amount of time for work. (Not too much and not too little.) As a family, we also did some traveling.

For Business

Los Angeles – Teach American Institute of Certified Public Accountants (AICPA) Course
San Francisco - Teach AICPA Course
Seattle - Teach AICPA Course
San Juan - Teach AICPA Course
Pittsburgh -Teach AICPA Course
Voorhees, NJ -Teach AICPA Course
Boston – Peer Review of other KPMG offices
Chicago – Peer Review
Davenport - Peer Review
Orlando – Peer Review
Miami - Peer Review of another CPA firm's office
Long Island City – Peer Review
C. W. Post College – Training
Dallas - Training
Atlanta - Training
New York City - Training
San Antonio – Training
Las Vegas (2 times) –Training and AICPA speech
Orlando (We have had our KPMG International Partners' meetings at the Orlando Marriott World Center almost every year that I was a Partner. Because of client deadlines, I only went to about 15 (out of 25) of these meetings. I have also attended 2 Retired Partners' meetings in Orlando since my retirement.)
Columbus, OH – Governmental Accounting Standards Board (GASB)
Cleveland, OH – GASB
New Orleans, LA – GASB
Philadelphia – various meetings

I never went outside the United States for business.
Travel to conferences
Charleston – National Association of State Auditors, Comptrollers, and Treasurers (NASACT)
Pittsburgh - NASACT
Louisville - NASACT & National Association of Accountants (NAA)
St. Louis – NAA
Pennsylvania Institute of CPAs
Philadelphia
Hilton Head
Orlando – Disney Boardwalk Hotel
National Pasta Association
Phoenix
Christian Business Men's Connection
Amelia Island
Atlanta
The Homestead in West Virginia
Gettysburg
Orlando – World Conference
Maritime Conference Center in Baltimore
Lancaster - Host
Vacations
Cross country family trip in the Chevy Suburban in 1971
Montego Bay, Jamaica
Palmas Del Mar, Puerto Rico
Las Vegas
Sanibel Island
Plymouth Rock, MA
Boston - Britt's 16th birthday
San Antonio - Kelly's 16th birthday
Orlando (numerous times)
Phoenix and California, Hoover Dam, Grand Canyon, Knott's Berry Farm - to visit Terri's friend, Wanda

Egypt - with Sherif Ettefa
Juarez, Mexico - 2 mission trips
Palm Coast, Florida - 3 times
Outer Banks, North Carolina – (approximately 20 times)

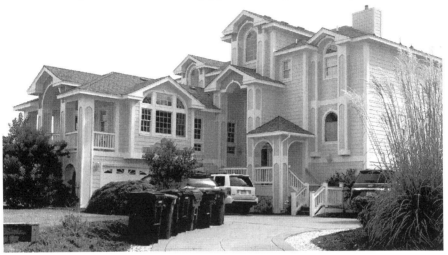

Duck, NC

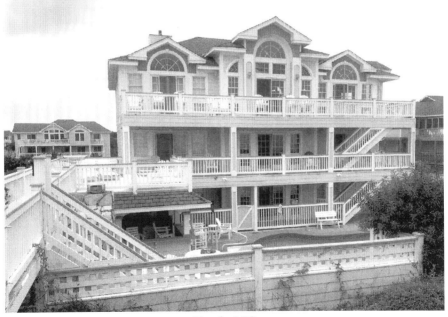

Duck, NC

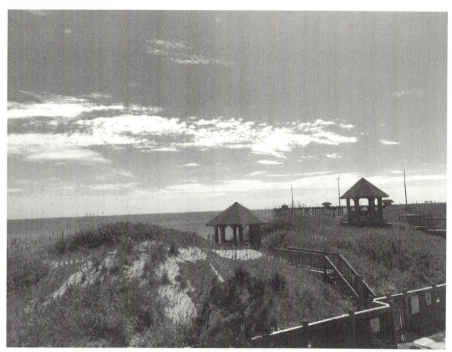
Nag's Head, NC

Grand Cayman Island - 2 times
Saint Croix
Toledo, OH - 2 times
New York City – several times

Several times, we spent some time in Williamsburg, VA on the way to the Outer Banks in North Carolina.

One of the traditions that we had at our annual Outer Banks trip was to do the "Lowering of the Basket." I would have the basket filled with sandwiches and drinks in the kitchen on the upper floor. I would lower the basket, with a rope, down to the pool area where the kids could enjoy the food.

We would play family games almost every year, including the games "Mafia" and "Wizard."

Another yearly tradition has been to take numerous family pictures on "Picture Night." When we started in 2002, we had three grandchildren and two sons-in-law. Now, we have 18 grandchildren, five sons-in-law, and a total of 30 people in our immediate family. God has truly blessed us.

My first airplane flight was from New York to Chicago in the summer of 1977. I went to a Peat Marwick government accounting and auditing training course with Dave Simon. I was 22 years old.

Worldwide Pandemic of 2020

Starting in January 2020, a global pandemic began with something called the Coronavirus or Covid 19.

Some people think that it was brought from China to the uttermost parts of the world. Some believe that China knew about it, and people were flying worldwide before they told the rest of the world.

This resulted in the shutdown of all "nonessential" businesses, sporting events, church gatherings, and any events that had more than a certain number of people. This has also led to the shutting down of Disney World and Disneyland, the casinos in Las Vegas and Atlantic City, gyms, restaurants, cruises, barbershops, and hairdressers. This was a worldwide event. Most of the other countries also "shut down." This also has led to no handshakes, people wearing facemasks, people washing their hands frequently, using hand sanitizer, and social distancing, which means standing 6 feet away from other people.

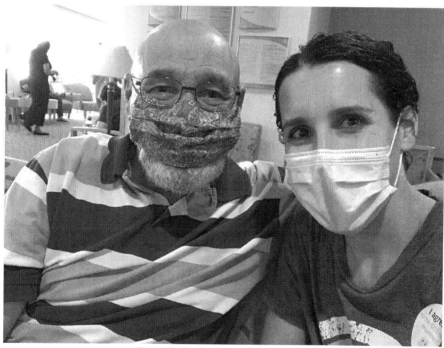

Dan & Brittany with masks

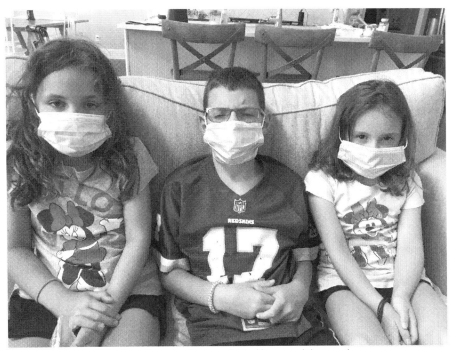

Blythe, Stevie Jr., and Colleen with masks

Grocery stores, food suppliers, and restaurants were considered "essential." However, most restaurants and fast food places had drive-up and/or pick-up only.

Several months later, businesses are opening slowly. However, large sporting events are only broadcasted on the TV with very few people attending in person.

Church services were only "live-streamed" for a while, but many have reopened and took certain precautions.

This led to putting doctors and nurses and other healthcare workers at significant risk to help those that came down with the virus. People are actively working on a vaccine to prevent this virus in the future. Many companies have reinvented themselves to make respirators and other Covid 19-related necessities. There is a shortage of hand sanitizer right now. Many things are in shortage right now.

Many locations were retrofitted to deal with this pandemic. For example, medical tents were set up in New York City in Central Park.

There were also conference centers throughout the United States that were retrofitted to become temporary hospitals. The two major medical ships that are owned by the United States government (the Comfort ship and the Mercy ship) were sent to New York City and Los Angeles for coronavirus patients.

Most of the bigger cities were hit harder with the virus than the smaller cities. Many people got sick and died from the coronavirus. By December 2020, over 16 million people got ill, and approximately 300,000 people died in the United States. The 1918 Spanish influenza pandemic also resulted in great tragedy. A book by John Barry titled The Great Influenza tells about the 1918 worldwide influenza.

This has led me to remain in Florida. My original plans were to be a "snowbird" in Florida from January through March 2020. However, I do not feel safe getting on an airplane to fly back to Pennsylvania because this virus is spread so quickly, and it can be contagious even though the other person that has the disease does not show signs of it for five days. Our dog, Tati, the black and white cockapoo, has been in Florida the whole time. She loves it in Florida.

In order to conduct meetings with other people for business and pleasure, many people were introduced to a relatively new computer system called Zoom (a conferencing software package).

Many people did remain working; however, they worked from home using Zoom for meetings.

Although I am retired, I use Zoom for:
- CBMC Mechanicsburg meetings on Monday mornings at 6:30 AM,
- Harrisburg Lions Club meetings on Tuesday at 7 PM,
- Waypoint Church Men's Bible Study on Wednesday at 7 PM,
- Several M28 Ministry board of director's meetings,
- Waypoint Church prayer meetings on Fridays at 8 AM.

This pandemic is a real indication of the power of God. No politician could have closed the whole world like this in a very short period of time.

This also led to quite a bit of economic instability. Unemployment in the United States hit record highs because people were no longer working. The federal government went into further debt (several trillion dollars) in order to send almost every citizen a "stimulus check" during the pandemic.

In some countries, for example, Nepal and countries in Africa, the pandemic prevented food from getting to the people, and there was actual concern about starvation.

The coronavirus's symptoms are a high fever, weakness, loss of taste and smell, and lung pain.

The President of the United States formed a committee led by Vice President Mike Pence to address this pandemic as it affects the United States. Additionally, the President was giving daily updates as to the number of sicknesses and deaths as well as the steps that the United States was taking to address this crisis.

This also led to a jigsaw puzzle shortage, a surge in the purchase of home exercise equipment, a rapid increase in Zoom use, and the cancelation of many events.

Many funny memes, stories, and jokes resulted from this pandemic. One of these follows:

"These times reminded me when I was a teenager; gas is cheap, and I'm grounded."

This pandemic has also led to having a National Prayer meeting sponsored by CBMC in September. It also led to the 2020 Prayer March in Washington DC led by Franklin Graham in late September.

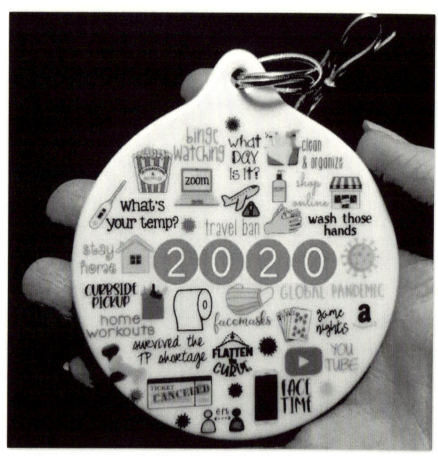
🎄 2020 Annual Events Christmas Ornament
💥 Sums up 2020 and hope to be even better next year! 🖤 Get it here 👉 https://bit.ly/380wdC4

Appendix 1
Spinocerebellar Ataxia

From Wikipedia, the free encyclopedia. 11/30/2020 2:15 PM Other names Spinocerebellar atrophy or Spinocerebellar degeneration

Spinocerebellar ataxia (SCA) is a progressive, degenerative, genetic disease with multiple types, each of which could be considered a neurological condition in its own right. An estimated 150,000 people in the United States have a diagnosis of spinocerebellar ataxia at any given time. SCA is hereditary, progressive, degenerative, and often fatal. There is no known effective treatment or cure. SCA can affect anyone of any age. The disease is caused by either a recessive or dominant gene. In many cases people are not aware that they carry a relevant gene until they have children who begin to show signs of having the disorder.

Signs and symptoms

Spinocerebellar ataxia (SCA) is one of a group of genetic disorders characterized by slowly progressive incoordination of gait and is often associated with poor coordination of hands, speech, and eye movements. A review of different clinical features among SCA subtypes was recently published describing the frequency of non-cerebellar features, like parkinsonism, chorea, pyramidalism, cognitive impairment, peripheral neuropathy, seizures, among others.[3] As with other forms of ataxia, SCA frequently results in atrophy of the cerebellum,[4] loss of fine coordination of muscle movements leading to unsteady and clumsy motion, and other symptoms.

The symptoms of an ataxia vary with the specific type and with the individual patient. In many cases a person with ataxia retains full mental capacity but progressively loses physical control.[citation needed]

Cause

The hereditary ataxias are categorized by mode of inheritance and causative gene or chromosomal locus. The hereditary ataxias can be inherited in an autosomal dominant, autosomal recessive, or X-linked manner.[citation needed]

Many types of autosomal dominant cerebellar ataxias for which specific genetic information is available are now known. Synonyms for autosomal-dominant cerebellar ataxias (ADCA) used prior to the current understanding of the molecular genetics were Marie's ataxia, inherited olivopontocerebellar atrophy, cerebello-olivary atrophy, or the more generic term "spinocerebellar degeneration." (Spinocerebellar degeneration is a rare inherited neurological disorder of the central nervous system characterized by the slow degeneration of certain areas of the brain. There are three forms of spinocerebellar degeneration: Types 1, 2, 3. Symptoms begin during adulthood.)[citation needed]

There are five typical autosomal-recessive disorders in which ataxia is a prominent feature: Friedreich ataxia, ataxia-telangiectasia, ataxia with vitamin E deficiency, ataxia with oculomotor apraxia (AOA), spastic ataxia. Disorder subdivisions: Friedreich's ataxia, Spinocerebellar ataxia, Ataxia telangiectasia, Vasomotor ataxia, Vestibulocerebellar, Ataxiadynamia, Ataxiophemia, Olivopontocerebellar atrophy, and Charcot-Marie-Tooth disease.[citation needed]

There have been reported cases where a polyglutamine expansion may lengthen when passed down, which often can result in an earlier age-of-onset and a more severe disease phenotype for individuals who inherit the disease allele. This falls under the category of genetic anticipation.[5] Several types of SCA are characterized by repeat expansion of the trinucleotide sequence CAG in DNA that encodes a polyglutamine repeat tract in protein. The expansion of CAG repeats over successive generations appears to be due to slipped strand mispairing during DNA replication or DNA repair.[6]

There are numerous types of autosomal-dominant cerebellar ataxias

There are five typical autosomal recessive disorders in which ataxia is a prominent feature

Medication

There is no cure for spinocerebellar ataxia, which is currently considered to be a progressive and irreversible disease, although not all types cause equally severe disability.[22]

In general, treatments are directed towards alleviating symptoms, not the disease itself. Many patients with hereditary or idiopathic forms of ataxia have other symptoms in addition to ataxia. Medications or other therapies might be appropriate for some of these symptoms, which could include tremor, stiffness, depression, spasticity, and sleep disorders, among others. Both onset of initial symptoms and duration of disease are variable. If the disease is caused by a polyglutamine trinucleotide repeat CAG expansion, a longer expansion may lead to an earlier onset and a more radical progression of clinical symptoms. Typically, a person afflicted with this disease will eventually be unable to perform daily tasks (ADLs).[23] However, rehabilitation therapists can help patients to maximize their ability of self-care and delay deterioration to certain extent.[24] Researchers are exploring multiple avenues for a cure including RNAi and the use of Stem Cells and several other avenues.[25]

On January 18, 2017 BioBlast Pharma announced completion of Phase 2a clinical trials of their medication, Trehalose, in the treatment of SCA3. BioBlast has received FDA Fast Track status and Orphan Drug status for their treatment. The information provided by BioBlast in their research indicates that they hope this treatment may prove efficacious in other SCA treatments that have similar pathology related to PolyA and PolyQ diseases.[26][27]

In addition, Dr. Beverly Davidson has been working on a methodology using RNAi technology to find a potential cure for over 2 decades.[28] Her research began in the mid-1990s and progressed to work with mouse models about a decade later and most recently has moved to a study with non-human primates. The results from her most recent research "are supportive of clinical application of this gene therapy".[29] Dr. Davidson along with Dr. Pedro Gonzalez-Alegre are currently working to move this technique into a Phase 1 clinical trial.

Finally, another gene transfer technology discovered in 2011 has also been shown by Dr. Davidson to hold great promise and offers yet another avenue to a potential future cure.[30]

N-Acetyl-Leucine[edit]

N-Acetyl-Leucine is an orally administered, modified amino acid that is being developed as a novel treatment for multiple rare and common neurological disorders by IntraBio Inc (Oxford, United Kingdom).[31]

N-Acetyl-Leucine has been granted multiple orphan drug designations from the U.S. Food & Drug Administration (FDA)[32] and the European Medicines Agency (EMA)[33] for the treatment of various genetic diseases, including Spinocerebellar Ataxias. N-Acetyl-Leucine has also been granted Orphan Drug Designations in the US and EU for the related inherited cerebellar ataxia Ataxia-Telangiectasia U.S. Food & Drug Administration (FDA)[34] and the European Medicines Agency (EMA).[35]

Published case series studies have demonstrated the effects of acute treatment with N-Acetyl-Leucine for the treatment of inherited cerebellar ataxias, including Spinocerebellar Ataxias.[36][37] These studies further demonstrated that the treatment is well tolerated, with a good safety profile.

A multinational clinical trial investigating N-Acetyl-L-Leucine for the treatment of a related inherited cerebellar ataxia, Ataxia-Telangiectasia, began in 2019.[38]

IntraBio is also conducting parallel clinical trials with N-Acetyl-L-Leucine for the treatment of Niemann-Pick disease type C[39] and GM2 Gangliosidosis (Tay-Sachs and Sandhoff Disease).[40] Future opportunities to develop N-Acetyl-Leucine include Lewy Body Dementia,[41]Amyotrophic lateral sclerosis, Restless Leg Syndrome, Multiple Sclerosis, and Migraine[42]

Rehabilitation

Physical therapists can assist patients in maintaining their level of independence through therapeutic exercise programs. One recent research report demonstrated a gain of 2 SARA points (Scale for the Assessment and Rating of Ataxia) from physical therapy.[43] In general, physical therapy emphasizes postural balance and gait training for ataxia patients.[44] General conditioning such as range-of-motion exercises and muscle strengthening would also be included in therapeutic exercise programs. Research showed that spinocerebellar ataxia 2 (SCA2) patients [45] with a mild stage of the disease gained significant improvement in static balance and neurological indices after six months of a physical therapy exercise training program.[46] Occupational therapists may assist patients with incoordination or ataxia issues through the use of adaptive devices. Such devices may include a cane, crutches, walker, or wheelchair for those with impaired gait. Other devices are available to assist with writing, feeding, and self-care if hand and arm coordination are impaired. A randomized clinical trial revealed that an intensive rehabilitation program with physical and occupational therapies for patients with degenerative cerebellar diseases can significantly improve functional gains in ataxia, gait, and activities of daily living. Some level of improvement was shown to be maintained 24 weeks post-treatment.[47] Speech language pathologists may use both behavioral intervention strategies as well as augmentative and alternative communication devices to help patients with impaired speech.

Appendix 2
TOC Funny Stories Chapter

Easter	50
Ted Williams Tunnel Dedication	51
Mobster Story	51
Dental Patient	52
Taco Bell Story	52
Expert Speaker	52
Small Gift	53
Discolored Plant	53
Dr. Sarosi	54
Washington DC Cab Ride	55
The Apostle Paul	56
Bond's Dock	56
The Book of Revelation	57
Highway Ride	57
Dinner Prayer	57
Clients	57
Glass of Water	58
The Idiot Book	58
Post Card	58
Egg Sandwiches	58
Rice	59

White Belt	59
Car Trip	59
Tesla Onesie	60
Assurance of Salvation	60
Yale University	60
Pops	61
Air Vent	62

Appendix 3
TOC Quotes Chapter

John Newton	101
Unknown	101
Grace Gems	101
Spurgeon	101
John Owen	101
Ruth Bell Graham	101
God's Not Dead 2	102
Martin Luther	102
Charles Spurgeon, Checkbook of Faith, 6/04	102
Thomas Manton, Works, 1:1 67-173	102
John Knox - speaking of the days during the Reformation	102
John Bunyan	102
Thomas Watson, Voices from The Past, Vol. 2, page 67	102
Richard Baxter, Voices from The Past, Vol. 1, p. 311	102

Appendix 4
CBMC Article

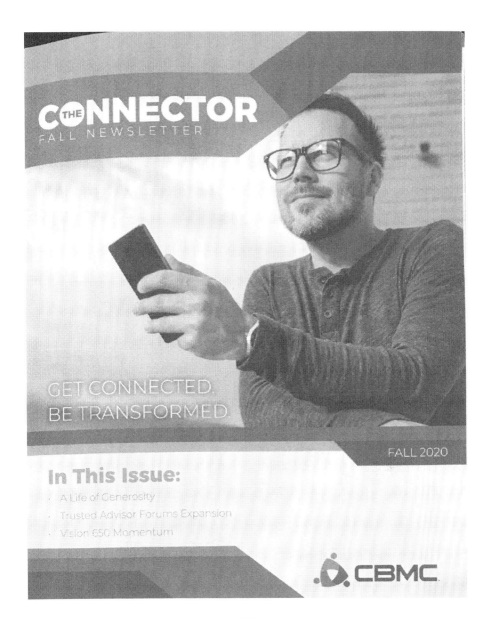

DAN KOVLAK: BEING INTRODUCED TO CBMC WAS 'TREMENDOUS' FROM THE START

Dan Kovlak was in his 40s, with a number of years experience as an auditor with a major CPA firm, when he first heard about CBMC. In 1999, while serving on the board of directors for Bethesda Mission, he attended a meeting where Charlie "Tremendous" Jones was speaking. Jones, a popular motivational speaker, CBMC member, and author, spoke highly of CBMC during the meeting.

"Based on what Charlie said, I was intrigued, so I looked in the telephone book to see if there was a local chapter," he said. A CBMC group was meeting Tuesday mornings in Mechanicsburg, PA, and Kovlak became a regular attendee.

There he met a number of men who would become lifelong friends and role models, including Dave Balinski. "Over the years, I had met very few Christians in the work environment. Men like Dave demonstrated that faith could be integrated into our work."

The weekly CBMC meetings, along with one-on-one interactions with men in the group, reinforced Kovlak's vision for serving Christ in the workplace.

Over the years, work assignments took him to different cities, but he stayed in contact with Dave Balinski, a valued brother in the faith. He lived out the truth of Proverbs 27:17, "As iron sharpens iron, so one man sharpens another," as they spent time together over the years.

In 2007, when Balinski accepted a full-time staff role in the area with CBMC, Kovlak added a new form of involvement: Investing in the ministry financially.

"Over the years my wife, Terri, and I have been blessed to be able to support CBMC financially, especially the staff in our area. We view CBMC's full-time workers as local missionaries.

"Many of the people who show up at our CBMC meetings don't realize we have missionaries in our midst, working here in the United States. We need to support them – I view financial investment in a ministry like CBMC as a spiritual act. Some of my support is designated for specific individuals, but the rest I just ask our leaders to use where they think it is best for the ministry. I believe wherever it goes in CBMC, God is putting it to good use."

Kovlak recognizes that while staff people serve to lead and help grow the ministry, the work of evangelizing and discipling business and professional men for Christ is everyone's job.

"Another one of my favorite verses, 2 Corinthians 5:20, speaks to this: 'Therefore, we are ambassadors for Christ, God making His appeal through us. We implore you on behalf of Christ, be reconciled to God.'"

Upon retiring after a 37-year career with KPMG, Kovlak has engaged in Operation Timothy discipling relationships with a number of young men; one later became one of his sons-in-law. Several years ago, he attended the wedding ceremony of another man he was discipling.

"Right now I have one OT relationship that has been going on for about five years. I always say that I learn as much in these discipling relationships as my Christian brothers learn from me. I find the time

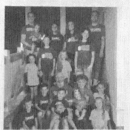

Dan and Terri Kovlak with their grandchildren

extremely gratifying."

Early this year, he went to Jacksonville, FL as a "snowbird" for a few months. When the COVID-19 pandemic hit, he found himself staying there much longer than expected. One of his Timothys wrote, "Dan, I just want to say I miss seeing you. When you get back to Pennsylvania, let's get back to having lunches together."

In Jacksonville, Kovlak attempted to start a CBMC group, inspired by the Vision 650 focus for planting new teams across the country. He met with members of several churches there, but the pandemic put plans for in-person meetings on hold indefinitely. However, he has been able to participate in meetings of his Connect3 team in Mechanicsburg via Zoom.

Today, the father of five daughters and 18 grandchildren (10 girls, seven boys, and one on the way), is also enjoying seeing his spiritual lineage grow through CBMC in a variety of ways, including Operation Timothy and his financial investments in the ministry.

HAVE A STORY TO SHARE? WE'D LOVE TO HEAR ABOUT WHAT GOD IS DOING IN YOUR AREA. EMAIL HMCAFEE@CBMC.COM.

Made in the USA
Middletown, DE
13 October 2022